Sleep Management in Nursing Practice

ity

9292

To Maureen, Calum, Ewan and Iain
KM

With great affection to Diane Closs and Betty and Bill Vaughan in the hope that they all master the art of sleeping
SJC

For Churchill Livingstone:

Senior Commissioning Editor: Alex Mathieson
Project Development Manager: Valerie Dearing
Project Manager: Jane Shanks

Sleep Management in Nursing Practice: An Evidence-Based Guide

Kevin Morgan BSc PhD

Director, Centre for Ageing and Rehabilitation Studies,
School of Health and Related Research, University of Sheffield, UK

S. José Closs BSc PhD MPhil RGN

Director of Research, Division of Nursing, School of Healthcare Studies,
University of Leeds, UK

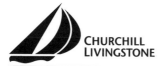

CHURCHILL
LIVINGSTONE

EDINBURGH LONDON NEW YORK PHILADELPHIA SYDNEY TORONTO

CHURCHILL LIVINGSTONE
An imprint of Harcourt Brace and Company Limited

© Harcourt Brace and Company Limited 1999

𝕯 is a registered trade mark of Harcourt Brace and Company Limited

The right of Kevin Morgan and S. José Closs to be identified as authors of this work has been asserted by them in accordance with the Copyright, Designs, and Patents Act 1988.

First published 1999

ISBN 0 443 05701 X

British Library Cataloguing in Publication Data
A catalogue record for this book is available from the British Library.

Library of Congress Cataloging in Publication Data
A catalog record for this book is available from the Library of Congress.

Although every effort has been made to chase copyright owners of illustrations, if any have inadvertently been missed the publisher will be happy to insert the appropriate acknowledgement at the first opportunity.

Note
Medical knowledge is constantly changing. As new information becomes available, changes in treatment, procedures, equipment and the use of drugs become necessary. The authors and the publishers have, as far as it is possible, taken care to ensure that the information given in this text is accurate and up-to-date. However, readers are strongly advised to confirm that the information, especially with regard to drug usage, complies with the latest legislation and standards of practice.

The
publisher's
policy is to use
**paper manufactured
from sustainable forests**

Printed in China

Contents

Preface

Insomnia affects approximately one in ten otherwise healthy adults. It is a frequently encountered adjunct to ill-health, life events, and trauma; and it is a major source of public expenditure both when treated, and when untreated. Yet insomnia remains poorly understood by many health care professionals who regularly encounter both the complaint and the consequences of chronic sleep disturbance.

The reasons for this are partly historical. One of the more subtle 'side-effects' of hypnotic drugs is that they have helped to define, narrowly and perhaps unfairly, who should take responsibility for poor sleep. Since the introduction of effective sleep medication, insomnia has tended to be seen, both by patients and by many professionals, as the responsibility of prescribing doctors. In recent years, however, the momentum of sleep disorders medicine, the eclecticism of contemporary sleep research, and the continued development of effective psychological treatments have clearly demonstrated that insomnia management benefits from multidisciplinary attention. It is the overall aim of this book, therefore, to encourage a broader clinical ownership of insomnia, and to facilitate an effective nursing contribution to the management of problem sleep.

Because the issues considered here tend to be, at best, scattered (but at worst, ignored) in the nursing literature, the content and organisation of the book reflect three further aims. First, to provide the practising nurse with a source reference on basic aspects of human sleep and its measurement. Second, to provide an accessible, but adequately detailed introduction to the nature and causes of insomnia. And third, to provide an evidence-based overview of current treatment options, and a framework for their delivery.

To meet these aims, information is presented in a sequence which, chapter by chapter, develops the themes of sleep and insomnia management. Most chapters have a stand-alone quality, and may be read in isolation. If, however, you are professionally interested in optimising the sleep quality of patients, and if you lack direct experience and think that this book may be of value, then our advice to you is the same as that offered to the White Rabbit by the King of Hearts: 'Begin at the beginning, and go on till you come to the end: then stop'.

Encouraging a broader responsibility for identifying and managing insomnia will, of course, require some adjustment in professional attitudes, boundaries and practices. The potential benefits to the patient, however, are considerable. It is hoped that ultimately, the recognition and effective management of sleep problems will find a permanent place in both the pre- and post-registration education and training of nurses, and all professional carers.

1999
                                        Kevin Morgan
                                        S. José Closs

Acknowledgements

We are grateful to Winslow Press and Chapman and Hall for allowing material from earlier books to be reproduced here. Thanks also to the staff and postgraduate students of the Centre for Ageing and Rehabilitation Studies, who helped provide space for the completion of this book. Finally, special thanks to Ann Hilton for her support throughout the preparation of the manuscript.

Sleep in nursing practice

Learning outcomes

This chapter introduces the topics of sleep and sleep disorders and places the management of disturbed sleep into a nursing context. On completing this chapter you should be able to:

- provide three reasons why nurses should know about sleep
- describe a sleep cycle
- define three diagnostic criteria for insomnia
- distinguish between primary and secondary insomnias
- recognise some of the limitations in your own knowledge of sleep.

INTRODUCTION
Why should nurses know about sleep?

In nursing, sleep has always mattered. Florence Nightingale, for example, not only emphasised the role of the nurse in promoting sleep, but described the *maintenance* of sound sleep as 'a *sine qua non* of all good nursing' (Nightingale 1859). Yet it would not be an exaggeration to suggest that, at the present time, those with insomnia do not get the best out of contemporary health care systems. Some 130 years after Nightingale prioritised sleep in her *Notes on Nursing*, an editorial in *The Lancet* concluded that, within the Health Service, complaints of poor sleep continue to attract responses 'unstructured by medical education and uninfluenced by developments in clinical sleep research' (Anonymous 1991). While these comments could still be applied equally to both medical and nursing practice, the situation is certainly set to change.

Once the province of common sense and experience, the nursing management of sleep is increasingly being recognised as an important area for research, education and evidence-based training. Most comprehensive nursing textbooks now include some information on disorders of sleep. The clinical, managerial and occupational issues relating to hospital nursing at night are also receiving increased attention (McMahon 1992). Within this context of a growing emphasis on evidence-based practice and rapid developments in clinical sleep research, it is now possible to identify at least five straightforward reasons why nurses should be more aware of sleep and its disorders. First, in both community and hospital settings, the nurse is frequently the first health care professional to encounter either the complaint of insomnia or the consequences of protracted sleep loss. Second, as a sensitive index of health and psychological well-being, changes in sleep represent an important, and measurable, outcome of nursing practice. Third, nurses are often well placed to control the sleeping environment and improve or maintain sleep quality. Fourth, research into the causes and treatment of insomnia has, in recent years, identified a number of therapies, strategies and techniques for assessing and effectively treating the patient with insomnia. While rarely deployed in nursing practice, many of these approaches complement or extend the existing skills of the post-registration nurse. And finally, there is an important need to recognise the emergence and continued development of sleep disorders medicine as both a specialised area of research and an increasingly specialised area of nursing and medical practice. Since many nurses will be unfamiliar with the constructs and vocabulary of sleep medicine this chapter introduces two topics fundamental to an understanding of sleep management: the nature of normal sleep and the symptoms of sleep disorders. The quiz at the end of the chapter then draws attention to the relevance of these and other aspects of sleep in nursing practice.

NORMAL SLEEP AND DISORDERS OF SLEEP
What is normal sleep?

There is an old, and possibly apocryphal story told in geriatric medicine about an elderly man who complains to the family doctor of discomfort in his knee. The doctor is sympathetic, but comments that, in advanced age, it is not unusual to have a stiff and painful knee joint. At this, the patient points out, with some irritation, that his other knee is the same age, but does not hurt a bit. These two views of normality, one based on individual experience and the other based on population expectations, have a particular significance when judging the normality of sleep. Sleep, like pain, can be intimate and socially inconspicuous. Most of us know what our 'normal' sleep feels like. Deviations from this norm, periods of disturbed or poor quality sleep, are as recognisable to us as they are unwelcome. Nevertheless, sleep itself also possesses a 'normal' structure, with individuals tending to show sleeping patterns typical (i.e. normal) for their gender, age group or culture. Importantly, then, both views are valid. And since both of these aspects of sleep are combined in the assessment and in the understanding of insomnia, both will be considered here.

The EEG structure of sleep

Since the discovery of rapid eye movement (REM) sleep in the early 1950s (Aserinsky & Kleitman 1953), the electroencephalogram (EEG), combined with recordings of eye movements (the electro-oculogram or EOG) and chin muscle tone (the electromyogram or EMG), has provided the standard tool for exploring the structure of human sleep. In 1968, internationally agreed criteria for interpreting the 'polysomnogram' (i.e. the EEG, EOG, and EMG recordings made during sleep) were published (Rechtschaffen & Kales 1968). These criteria, incorporating the accumulated wisdom of 40 years of brain-wave recording, remain in use today, and describe five 'stages' of sleep (Fig. 1.1).

When relaxed (but with the eyes closed) the EEG is characterised by alpha waves, mixed voltage activity with a frequency of 8–13 cycles per second. Stage 1 sleep, drowsiness, is accompanied by lower voltage mixed frequency activity which may appear haphazard or 'desynchronised' or may be regular and 'synchronised' at about 4–6 cycles per second. The onset of light sleep is determined by the appearance of stage 2, mixed voltage activity of the alpha type showing clear episodes of 12–14 cycles per second 'sleep spindles'. Stages 3 and 4 accompany 'deep sleep', and are frequently subsumed within the single term 'slow wave sleep' or SWS. These slow waves are of high voltage, with a frequency of between 1–4 cycles per second, the slower and more uniformly high voltage pattern being characteristic of stage 4. The EEG of

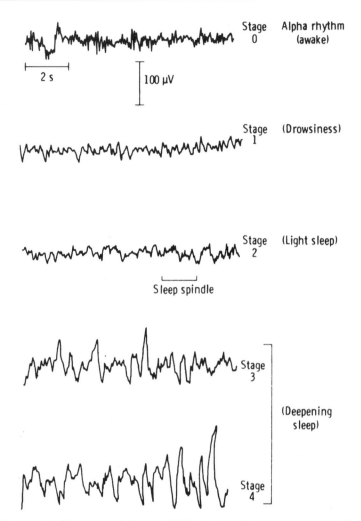

Figure 1.1 Electroencephalogram (EEG) tracings of sleep stages recorded from a young adult.

rapid eye movement or REM sleep is similar to that of stage 1. However, unlike any other sleep stage, it is also accompanied by episodic rapid eye movements and profound relaxation of the muscles which maintain posture (the so-called antigravity muscles of the limbs and trunk), both being events clearly visible on the EOG and EMG traces (it is for this reason that REM sleep earned the epithet 'paradoxical sleep', since the EEG shows arousal, while the EOG and EMG show relaxation). REM sleep is also accompanied by phases of quite intense physiological activity: the pulse rate quickens, blood pressure rises, respiration rates increase, and oxygen consumption is higher than at any other time during sleep. And finally, the REM stage is closely linked to dreaming. In experimental studies with young adults, over 80% of REM awakenings are associated with the recall of vivid, narrative dreams. Non-REM awakenings, on the other hand, are associated with lower levels of dream recall, or no dream recall at all (Dement & Kleitman 1957).

A typical laboratory analysis of sleep involves the continuous recording of EEG, EOG, and EMG from the onset of sleep to final awakening. The resulting record is interpreted or 'scored' using the criteria outlined above. The order and duration of each sleep stage is calculated, and the frequency of shifts from one stage to another computed. A convenient way of graphically representing the structure of a single sleep period is shown in Figure 1.2. The time spent in each stage is represented by horizontal lines, while the vertical lines indicate a shift from one stage to another. (In reality, these shifts are a little less abrupt than Fig. 1.2 suggests.) Clearly the five sleep stages follow each other in a cyclical fashion. Having progressed through stages 1 to 4 (non-REM or NREM stages), an individual may then return, stepwise to stage 2 before the first REM period begins, after which the same cycle starts again. Measurements of sleep which are commonly derived from the all-night polysomnogram are summarised in Box 1.1.

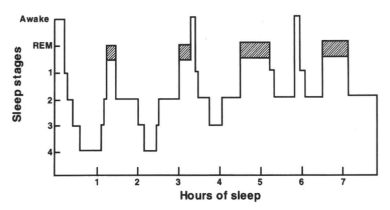

Figure 1.2 Hypnogram for a typical young adult. Horizontal lines represent time spent in each stage of sleep; vertical lines indicate transitions between sleep stages. Shaded areas indicate periods of REM sleep.

Box 1.1 Measurements of sleep derived from the all-night polysomnogram (EEG, EOG and EMG)

Sleep onset latency (SOL). The time taken from the decision to go to sleep (or, in the laboratory, from 'lights out') to the appearance of the first stage of actual sleep (stage 2).

Sleep period time (SPT). The time from sleep onset to final awakening.

Wakefulness after sleep onset (WASO) or intervening wakefulness. Episodes of (usually 30 seconds or more) stage 0 that occur within the sleep period. Intervening wakefulness can be expressed in terms of *duration* (e.g. total minutes of wakefulness) or *frequency* (e.g. number of awakenings per night). In either case, wakefulness of this type indicates the degree of sleep disturbance.

Frequency of stage shifts. Transitions from one sleep stage to another are referred to as stage shifts, and are frequently associated with gross body movements. The number of shifts observed during the sleep period can also be used as a measure of sleep disturbance.

Total sleep time (TST). This refers to the period from sleep onset to final awakening (i.e. the sleep period) minus any intervening wakefulness. Because periods of significant wakefulness are deducted, total sleep time is a rather pure measure of the actual duration of sleep.

Duration of each sleep stage. The time spent in each sleep stage during a single night can be expressed either in units of time (e.g. total minutes of stage 1, etc.) or as a percentage, usually of the sleep period time (this allows for the calculation of the percentage of intervening wakefulness).

Time in bed (TIB). While fairly meaningless in laboratory situations where the times of going to and getting out of bed are frequently imposed, the time spent in bed becomes particularly important when individuals are permitted to 'free run' and select their own time of arising. Time in bed is usually defined as the period from 'lights out' (i.e. settling down to sleep) to rising.

Sleep efficiency. The ratio of time in bed to total sleep time, usually expressed as:

$$(\text{Total sleep time} \div \text{Time in bed}) \times 100$$

is frequently used as an indication of sleep efficiency. This measurement assumes that if someone is in bed, then he or she is at least *trying* to get to sleep.

Measuring depth of sleep

The polysomnogram also provides some insight into the quality of sleep likely to be reported by the sleeper. The number of stage shifts, for example, (see Fig. 1.2) indicates to some extent the degree of restlessness during sleep. A typically restless night would involve many such changes from one sleep stage to another. Polysomnographic methods can also provide insights into the *depth* of sleep.

Most people appreciate the metaphor of 'deep' sleep, it refers to sleep from which we are not easily aroused. One of the many differences between the sleep stages described above is their depth, as measured by the minimum amount of noise required to wake the sleeping person (a measurement called the auditory awakening threshold or AAT). The intensity of an auditory tone required to wake a sleeping experimental subject, for example, is greatest in stage 4, slightly less in stage 3, and least in stage 2 (see, for example, Busby et al 1994, Zepelin et al 1984). REM sleep presents a rather special case, but in terms of the auditory awakening threshold, is at least as 'deep' as stage 4. It is for this reason that individuals are more, or less, easily awakened at different times in the night.

Sleep and the circadian rhythm

Both the need to, and the occurrence of sleep are regulated by a biological clock with a periodicity of about 24 hours – the circadian rhythm (circadian means 'around the day'). Viewed in this way, sleep is not an isolated event, but rather forms part of a sleep–wake *cycle* synchronised with the changing patterns of day and night. Of course, the biological clock can be reset (as, for example, when mechanical clocks are moved forwards and backwards in the spring and autumn, or following time-zone changes in travel). But this 'entrainment' can take a little time. Under normal circumstances, sleep–wake and day/night synchronisation are maintained with what are called 'zeitgebers' (time givers), those rhythmic parts of our routine like meal times, work schedules, or light and dark. Other aspects of our physiology are also entrained to the 24-hour day, most noticeably temperature, which rises and falls by as much as a degree between early evening, and the small hours of the morning. While some forms of insomnia result from desynchronisation, most sleep disturbances can weaken links between zeitgebers and body clocks (as, for example occurs when night-time sleeplessness leads to habitual daytime naps). This relationship between sleep and waking behaviour is strongly emphasised in current criteria for insomnia (below).

Sleep structure and age

People of the same age may show wide individual differences in the characteristics of their normal sleep, with some requiring more or less sleep than others to function efficiently during the day. One of the most influential factors determining the structure of adult sleep, however, is age. With increasing age, from early adulthood to later life, sleep becomes progressively more fragmented, shorter and lighter. As we shall see in the next chapter, these changes have far-reaching implications for sleep quality, making age and ageing fundamental to an understanding of insomnia.

Sleep fragmentation. Relative to that of the young, the sleep of older people is characterised by more frequent 'shifts' from one sleep stage to another, and more frequent episodes of intervening wakefulness during the night (Fig. 1.3). Both events result in sleep which is more broken or fragmented. Throughout adult life, these 'spontaneous' nocturnal awakenings tend to be more common among men, a finding possibly related to the disturbing effects of nocturnal penile tumescence (NPT) which occurs quite mechanically during REM sleep in sexually non-dysfunctional men of all ages (Karacan et al 1975).

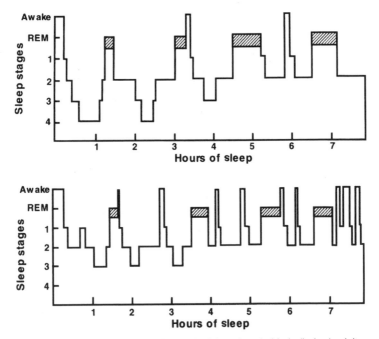

Figure 1.3 Typical hypnograms for young (above) and elderly (below) adults. Shaded areas indicate periods of REM sleep.

Duration of sleep. As periods of intervening wakefulness increase with age in both frequency and duration, the total time spent asleep at night shows a reciprocal decrease. As a result, sleep efficiency (time spent asleep divided by time spent in bed) also tends to decrease (see Bliwise 1993). One of the most consistently reported age-related structural changes within NREM sleep is the progressive reduction in EEG slow waves (those associated with stages 3 and 4 or slow wave sleep) and, for many people, the virtual disappearance of stage 4 altogether (Fig. 1.3).

Depth of sleep. With increasing age, depth of sleep appears to be affected both quantitatively and qualitatively. Changes in the architecture of sleep so far considered result in a diminution of deeper slow wave sleep (SWS), and a reciprocal increase in stages 2 (light sleep) and 1 (drowsiness). Older sleep is therefore *structurally* lighter. In addition, studies of auditory awakening thresholds show qualitative changes in the depth of individual sleep stages. It has been shown, for example, that during stages 2, 4, and REM, older people are more easily awakened by a given level of noise (i.e. have lower auditory awakening thresholds) than are younger people (Busby et al 1994, Zepelin et al 1984).

What are sleep disorders?

Problems associated with sleep quality and quantity, and conditions closely associated with the sleep cycle or the physiological mechanisms of sleep, are now collectively referred to as *sleep disorders*. From its origins in academic sleep laboratories (mainly in the USA), sleep medicine has developed rapidly in recent years. The revised International Classification of Sleep Disorders (ICSD; American Sleep Disorders Association 1990), for example, currently recognises three broad diagnostic classes which collectively subsume some 88 distinct sleep–wake irregularities. By far the most commonly reported, and commonly treated, complaints, however, are the disorders of initiating or maintaining sleep, or the insomnias. It is the insomnias which provide the focus for this book. In order to place these complaints in a broader context, and to explore some important aspects of disordered sleep, this section considers the way in which sleep disorders are currently classified, and how insomnia is currently defined.

Insomnia is now explicitly defined in three diagnostic systems: the International Classification of Diseases 10th edition (ICD-10) Classification of Mental and Behavioral Disorders (WHO 1993); the Diagnostic and Statistical Manual of Mental Disorders (DSM-IV; American Psychiatric Association 1994); and the International Classification of Sleep Disorders (ICSD; American Sleep Disorders Association 1990). While all three classifications largely agree on the symptoms of insomnia, there are important differences both in terminology and emphasis.

Diagnosing insomnia: ICD-10

ICD-10 broadly divides sleep disorders into organic and nonorganic (Fig. 1.4), with the latter category further subdivided into dyssomnias (disturbances of the amount, quality, or timing of sleep) and parasomnias (abnormal episodic events occurring during sleep, for example, sleepwalking, nightmares, etc.). In this system 'nonorganic insomnia', is a dyssomnia characterised by persistent (i.e. at least three times a week for at least 1 month) difficulty in getting to sleep or staying asleep (or poor quality sleep), which causes the individual concern, and markedly interferes with social or occupational functioning. ICD-10 does not explicitly discriminate between primary insomnia (where the sleep disturbance may be the *only* presenting condition) and secondary insomnia (where the sleep disturbance accompanies other physical or mental disorders).

Diagnosing insomnia: DSM-IV

DSM-IV uses a broader classification which recognises four main types of sleep disorder (Fig. 1.5): sleep disorders related to another mental disorder; sleep disorders due to a general medical condition; substance-induced sleep disorders; and primary sleep disorders (i.e. those not associated with a psychiatric, medical, or pharmacological cause). *Primary sleep disorders* in DSM-IV are analogous to the *nonorganic sleep disorders* of ICD-10, and are similarly divided into dyssomnias and parasomnias, with insomnia (as 'primary insomnia') again subsumed within the dyssomnias. In DSM-IV, the diagnostic features of primary insomnia are also similar to those described in ICD-10 and include a persistent (i.e. for at least 1 month) complaint of difficulty initiating or maintaining sleep (or of non-restorative sleep) which causes the individual 'significant' distress

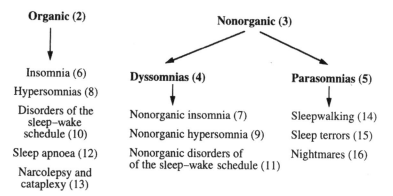

ICD-10: Sleep Disorders (1)*

Organic (2)

Insomnia (6)
Hypersomnias (8)
Disorders of the sleep–wake schedule (10)
Sleep apnoea (12)
Narcolepsy and cataplexy (13)

Nonorganic (3)

Dyssomnias (4)

Nonorganic insomnia (7)
Nonorganic hypersomnia (9)
Nonorganic disorders of of the sleep–wake schedule (11)

Parasomnias (5)

Sleepwalking (14)
Sleep terrors (15)
Nightmares (16)

*numbers in parentheses refer to ICD-10 definitions

Figure 1.4   Overview of sleep disorders as described in the International Classification of Diseases (ICD-10).
ICD-10 (sleep disorders): definitions
(Only a sample of definitions are provided here. For further information, see the source reference.)

(1)   Produced by the World Health Organization, the International Classification of Diseases, 10th edition (ICD-10), provides a diagnostic classification of diseases for epidemiological and health management purposes. While not primarily intended as a diagnostic manual, detailed diagnostic information is available in what are termed 'speciality-based adaptations' of the ICD.

(2, 3)   ICD-10 broadly divides sleep disorders into organic (Code G47-) and nonorganic (Code F51-). Organic sleep disorders are those arising from an identifiable physical cause. In ICD-10, these sleep disorders are listed under 'Diseases of the Nervous System' (Code G47). Nonorganic sleep disorders (Code F51-) may have emotional *or* physical origins; 'emotional causes are considered to be a primary factor'. Detailed diagnostic information on nonorganic sleep disorders is provided in *The ICD-10 Classification of Mental and Behavioural Disorders: Clinical Descriptions and Diagnostic Guidelines.* (World Health Organization 1993) which sub-divides nonorganic sleep disorders into dyssomnias and parasomnias.

(4)   In ICD-10, dyssomnia is defined as a primarily psychogenic condition in which the predominant disturbance is in the amount, quality or timing of sleep.

(5)   Parasomnias are abnormal episodic events which occur during sleep. In childhood, such events may be considered developmental (e.g. sleepwalking), while in adulthood they are mainly psychogenic.

(6)   Here the term *insomnia* refers to the disorders of initiating or maintaining sleep. In ICD-10, insomnia is described as a condition of unsatisfactory sleep quantity and/or quality which persists for a period of time. In ICD-10, organic insomnias result from identifiable physical disorders which can be classified elsewhere in the ICD system.

(7) The ICD-10 Classification of Mental and Behavioural Disorders describes four essential clinical features of nonorganic insomnia: (i) the complaint is either of difficulty falling asleep or maintaining sleep, or of poor quality of sleep; (ii) the sleep disturbance has occurred at least three times per week for at least 1 month; (iii) there is a preoccupation with the sleeplessness and excessive concern over its consequences at night and during the day; and (iv) the unsatisfactory quantity and/or quality of sleep either causes marked distress or interferes with social and occupational functioning.

(8, 9) Hypersomnia is defined in ICD-10 as a condition either of excessive daytime sleepiness and sleep attacks (not accounted for by an inadequate amount of sleep) or prolonged transition to the fully aroused state upon awakening. In ICD-10, organic hypersomnias result from identifiable physical disorders which can be classified elsewhere in the ICD system. In the absence of definite evidence of organic aetiology, however, hypersomnia, according to the ICD-10 Classification of Mental and Behavioural Disorders, is usually associated with mental disorders (e.g. recurrent depressive disorder, or a depressive episode, etc.).

(10, 11) ICD-10 defines disorders of the sleep–wake schedule as a lack of synchrony between the individual's sleep–wake schedule and the desired sleep–wake schedule for the environment, resulting in a complaint of either insomnia or hypersomnia. Distinguishing between organic and nonorganic disorders of the sleep–wake schedule can be difficult, and ICD-10 acknowledges that many such disturbances which originate biologically can have a strong psychological component on presentation. Shiftwork, and frequent trans-meridian travel are common causes.

(12) Sleep apnoea refers to a temporary cessation of breathing during sleep. This may be due to obstruction of the upper airway (obstructive sleep apnoea), or a loss of respiratory effort (central sleep apnoea). Mixed sleep apnoeas result from a combination of the two. The presenting symptom is often hypersomnolence.

(13) Narcolepsy refers to a neurological syndrome characterised by an abnormal irresistible sleep tendency where individuals may fall asleep quite abruptly for varying periods during the day.

(14) Sleepwalking (somnambulism), like night terrors, occurs during the deeper stages of sleep (stages 3 and 4), is more common in childhood, and tends to run in families. Typically, the sleepwalker arises from bed (usually during the first third of nocturnal sleep, and walks about, exhibiting low levels of awareness, reactivity and motor skill.

(15) Sleep terrors or night terrors are nocturnal episodes of terror and panic, with intense motility and vocalisation. Like sleepwalking, night terrors occur during the deeper stages of sleep (stages 3 and 4), are more common in childhood, and tend to run in families. The individual sits up, or gets up, with a panicky scream usually during the first third of nocturnal sleep. On awakening there is usually no recollection of the episode.

(16) Nightmares are dream experiences loaded with anxiety and fear, of which the individual has very detailed recall.

and is associated with impaired social or occupational functioning. Unlike ICD-10, however, DSM-IV taxonomically separates primary insomnia from those secondary insomnias associated with other disorders. Nevertheless, the system does recognise that, under some circumstances, distinguishing *primary insomnia* from *insomnia related to another mental disorder* 'can be especially difficult', and that *sleep disorders due to general medical conditions* are 'characterized by symptoms similar to those in primary sleep disorders'.

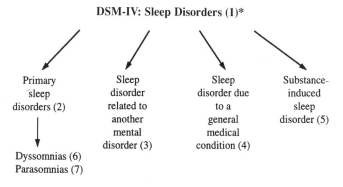

DSM-IV: Sleep Disorders (1)*

Primary sleep disorders (2)

Dyssomnias (6)
Parasomnias (7)

Sleep disorder related to another mental disorder (3)

Sleep disorder due to a general medical condition (4)

Substance-induced sleep disorder (5)

*numbers in parentheses refer to DSM-IV definitions

Figure 1.5   Overview of sleep disorders as described in the Diagnostic and Statistical Manual (4th edn) of the American Psychiatric Association (DSM-IV). *DSM-IV (sleep disorders): definitions*
(Only a sample of definitions are provided here. For further information, see the source reference.)

(1) Produced by the American Psychiatric Association, the 4th edition of the Diagnostic and Statistical Manual of Mental Disorders (DSM-IV) provides detailed criteria for the diagnosis and statistical coding of sleep disorders. In DSM-IV, sleep disorders are organised into four sections according to presumed aetiology: primary sleep disorders; sleep disorder related to another mental disorder; sleep disorder due to a general medical condition; and substance induced sleep disorder. All sections include insomnia-type disorders.

(2) Primary sleep disorders are assumed to arise from abnormalities in sleep–wake generating or timing mechanisms, often complicated by conditioning (i.e. learned) factors.

(3) Sleep disorder related to another mental disorder involves a prominent complaint of sleep disturbance that results from a diagnosable mental disorder, but is severe enough to warrant independent clinical attention.

(4) This category involves a prominent complaint of sleep disturbance that results from the direct physiological effects of a general medical condition on the sleep–wake system.

(5) Substance induced sleep disorder involves prominent complaints of sleep disturbance that result from the concurrent use, or recent discontinuation of use, of a substance (including medication).

(6) DSM IV defines dyssomnias as primary disorders of initiating or maintaining sleep, or of excessive sleepiness. Dyssomnias are characterised by a disturbance in the amount, quality, or timing of sleep. Primary insomnia is included in this category.

(7) Parasomnias are defined as disorders characterised by abnormal behavioural or physiological events occurring in association with sleep, specific sleep stages, or sleep–wake transitions.

Diagnosing insomnia: ICSD

The most detailed classification of sleep disorders is that provided by the ICSD (Fig. 1.6), which defines 12 subtypes of 'insomnia disorder' (i.e. disorders of initiating or maintaining sleep), and over 50 different insomnia syndromes. Since many of these diagnoses require specialised instrumental monitoring (often laboratory-based polysomnography) the value of the ICSD in everyday practice is probably limited. The commonest forms of insomnia recognised by this classification (and those closest to the 'nonorganic' and 'primary' insomnias of ICD-10 and DSM-IV) include *psychophysiological insomnia* (characterised by psychosomatic arousal, excessive concern about sleep adequacy, and somatised tension) *inadequate sleep hygiene* (where the sleep problem appears to be caused or maintained by maladaptive practices), and so-called *sleep-state misperception* (where the chronic complaint of insomnia is not 'corroborated' by polysomnographic findings). Though relatively rare, the ICSD diagnosis of *idiopathic insomnia* (a near lifelong constitutional predisposition to poor quality sleep) may also be regarded as a 'classic' insomnia.

Conclusions

Overall, then, ICD-10, DSM-IV, and ICSD show widespread consensus as to what constitutes an insomnia, with many apparent differences being terminological rather than fundamental (in each system, for example, the same clinical presentation could attract the diagnosis of 'organic insomnia', 'primary insomnia' or 'psychophysiological insomnia' respectively). In clinical field studies where all three systems have been used, diagnoses have been found to interrelate logically (Buysse et al 1994). While both the recognition and use of formal diagnostic systems for sleep disorders continues to grow, such categorisations remain rare in clinical practice. Nevertheless, if any one system were to be recommended for use at the present time, then DSM-IV would appear to be the system of choice since:

- it is already widely accepted as the diagnostic 'gold standard' in many areas of mental health
- it clearly presents insomnia as a mental health, physical health, and primary disorder
- it explicitly cross references its own diagnoses with those presented in ICSD.

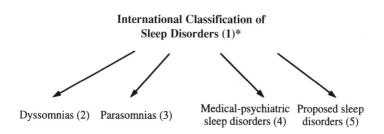

Figure 1.6 Overview of sleep disorders as described in the International Classification of Sleep Disorders (ICSD).
International Classification of Sleep Disorders (ICSD): definitions
(Only a sample of definitions are provided here. For further information, see the source reference.)

(1) The ICSD provides the most detailed classification of sleep–wake disorders, replacing the Diagnostic Classification of Sleep and Arousal Disorders published in 1979. Because of its detail, and the emphasis placed on electrophysiological recording to permit differential diagnosis, the ICSD system is probably unsuitable for use in most non-specialised care settings.

(2) In the ICSD, the dyssomnias include the disorders of initiating and maintaining sleep (the insomnias), and the disorders of excessive somnolence (the hypersomnias). Within the category *dyssomnia*, however, these disorders are divided into three major groups: intrinsic sleep disorders; extrinsic sleep disorders; and circadian rhythm sleep disorders.

(3) In the ICSD, parasomnias are defined as undesirable physical phenomena which occur predominantly during sleep, and are divided into four groups depending on the presenting phenomenology and their timing during sleep. These groups are: arousal disorders; sleep–wake transition disorders; parasomnias usually associated with REM sleep; and other parasomnias.

(4) Medical-psychiatric sleep disorders include those conditions 'commonly seen in the practice of sleep disorders medicine' (Thorpy 1994). This rather arbitrary category includes neurological, as well as medical and psychiatric illness.

(5) The ICSD continues to develop. The category of proposed sleep disorders includes those syndromes and conditions for which, at present, adequate substantiating information is unavailable.

A further important similarity in these diagnostic systems is the value each attaches to the individual's *experience* of sleep, and to the daytime consequences of sleep loss. Clearly, establishing either criterion requires some in-depth assessment. In reviewing and summarising current knowledge, this book aims specifically to raise levels of awareness, improve the assessment, and inform the nursing management of sleep and sleep disorders.

SLEEP IN NURSING PRACTICE
Assess your own knowledge

In order to provide a broad overview of those aspects of patient care which interact with the issues of sleep and insomnia, the quiz below tests your knowledge in a variety of different areas. The quiz has two objectives: first, to give you some feedback on what you do, or do not know about this subject; but second, and perhaps more importantly, to provide you with a clear idea of just how important, and useful, it is to be aware of sleep-related issues in nursing practice. Each item is evidence based, and is scored true or false. If you are interested in following up any of the points raised here, a 'starter' reference is provided with the answers. Incidentally, when adding up your score, remember that, on average, you could get 15/30 just by guessing!

Sleep quiz

Answer each item by recording 'True' or 'False' alongside the item number on a separate sheet. Score out of 30 (correct answers score 1; incorrect answers score 0).

1. After settling down for the night, healthy young adults take, on average, 10–15 minutes to fall asleep.
   True/False

2. Benzodiazepine hypnotics produce few noticeable withdrawal effects if discontinued after 3–4 weeks of continuous night-time usage.
   True/False

3. Poor sleep during a hospital stay is a rare problem for most inpatients.
   True/False

4. As people grow older they are more easily awakened by noise.
   True/False

5. Depressed people tend to sleep longer than non-depressed people.
   True/False

6. The duration of sleep increases during the week before the onset of labour.
   True/False

7. Sufferers of diabetes, epilepsy and chronic heart disease should be exempted from working night shifts.
   True/False

8. The propensity to snore is related to body weight.
   True/False

9. The strongest predictor of sudden infant death syndrome (SIDS) is leaving babies to sleep in a prone position.
   True/False

10. Between the ages of 6 and 10 years, the length of children's sleep increases.
    True/False

11. Peak growth hormone secretion occurs during slow wave sleep (SWS).
    True/False

12. Patients in intensive care units spend most of their time asleep.
    True/False

13. All healthy adults can learn to adjust to night-shift work with no ill-effects.
    True/False

14. Noise is the most common cause of sleep disruption in hospital.
    True/False

15. After settling down for the night, healthy elderly people take, on average, 5–10 minutes to fall asleep.
    True/False

16. The efficacy of benzodiazepine hypnotics declines with chronic use.
    True/False

17. Most complaints of poor sleep are made by people under the age of 50.
    True/False

18. Studies in which nurses' reports have been compared with EEG recordings show that nurses consistently underestimate the length of time their patients spend asleep.
    True/False

19. The prevalence of snoring increases with age among both men and women.
True/False

20. Beta adrenoceptor blockers ('beta-blockers') are a cause of restless and disturbed sleep.
True/False

21. Body temperature falls during sleep.
True/False

22. Benzodiazepine drugs used to treat anxiety can also be used as hypnotics.
True/False

23. Sleep disruption due to menopausal hot flushes can be successfully reduced by oestrogen therapy.
True/False

24. In general, increased levels of exercise during the day lead to improvements in the quality of sleep at night.
True/False

25. Those women in their second or subsequent pregnancy sleep worse than in their first pregnancy.
True/False

26. Most people need about 8 hours' sleep at night.
True/False

27. Malted milk drinks improve the quality of sleep.
True/False

28. Normal full-term babies spend about 20 hours asleep each day.
True/False

29. Sleepwalking is hereditary.
True/False

30. Women are more likely to complain of insomnia than are men.
True/False

Answers

1. *True.* See Williams R L et al 1974 Electroencephalography (EEG) of human sleep: clinical applications. John Wiley, New York.

2. *False.* See Adam K et al 1984 Effect of loprazalom and triazolam on sleep and overnight urinary cortisol. Psychopharmacology 82: 389–394.

3. *False.* See Closs S J 1992 Patients' night-time pain, analgesic provision and sleep after surgery. International Journal of Nursing Studies 29(4): 381–392.

4. *True.* See Zepelin H et al 1984 Effects of age on auditory awakening thresholds. Journal of Gerontology 39: 294–300.

5. *False.* See Reynolds C F, Kupfer D J, Houck P R, Hoch C C, Stack J A, Berman S R, Zimmer B 1988 Reliable discrimination of elderly depressed and demented patients by electroencephalographic sleep data. Archives of General Psychiatry 45: 258–264; and Kupfer D J, Ulrich R F, Coble P A et al 1985 Electroencephalographic sleep of younger depressives. Archives of General Psychiatry 42: 806–810.

6. *False.* See Evans M L, Dick M J, Clark A S 1995 Sleep during the week before labor: relationships to labor outcomes. Clinical Nursing Research 4(3): 238–249.

7. *True.* See Koller M 1989 Preventive health measures for shiftworkers. In: Wallace M (ed) Managing shiftwork. Brain Behaviour Research Institute, La Trobe University, Bundoora, Australia, pp. 17–24.

8. *True.* See Bliwise D L, Feldman D E, Bliwise N G et al 1987 Risk factors for sleep disordered breathing in heterogeneous geriatric populations. Journal of the American Geriatrics Society 35: 132–141.

9. *True.* See Fleming P J, Blair P S, Bacon C et al 1996 Environment of infants during sleep and risk of the sudden infant death syndrome: results of 1993–5 case-control study for confidential inquiry into still births and deaths in infancy. British Medical Journal 313: 191–195.

10. *False.* See Coble P A, Kupfer D J, Reynolds C F, Houck P 1987 EEG sleep of healthy children 6 to 12 years of age. In: Guilleminault C (ed) Sleep and its disorders in children. Raven Press, New York, pp. 32–33.

11. *True.* See Gronfier C, Luthringer R, Follenius M, Schaltenbrand N, Macher J P, Muzet A, Brandenberger G 1996 A quantitative evaluation of the relationships between growth hormone secretion and delta wave electroencephalographic activity during normal sleep and after enrichment in delta waves. Sleep 19: 817–824.

12. *False.* See Aurell J, Elmqvist D 1985 Sleep in the surgical intensive care unit: continuous polygraphic recording of sleep in nine patients receiving postoperative care. British Medical Journal 290: 1029–1032.

13. *False.* See Boivin D B, Czeisler C A, Dijk D J et al 1997 Complex interaction of the sleep–wake cycle and circadian phase modulates mood in healthy subjects. Archives of General Psychiatry 54: 145–152.

14. *True.* See Southwell M T, Wistow G 1995 Sleep in hospitals at night: are patients' needs being met? Journal of Advanced Nursing 21: 1101–1109.

15. *False.* See Webb W B 1982 Sleep in older persons: sleep structures in 50- to 60-year-old men and women. Journal of Gerontology 37: 581–586

16. *True.* See Lader M 1994 Benzodiazepines – a risk-benefit profile. CNS Drugs 1: 377–387.

17. *False.* See Ohayon M 1996 Epidemiologic study on insomnia in the general population. Sleep 19: S7–S15

18. *False.* See Weiss B L et al 1973 Once more, the inaccuracy of non-EEG estimates of sleep. American Journal of Psychiatry 130: 1282–1285.

19. *True.* See Lugarsi E et al 1980 Some epidemiological data on snoring and cardiovascular disturbance. Sleep 3: 221–224.

20. *True.* See Kostis J B, Rosen R C, Holzer B C et al 1990 CNS side effects of centrally-active antihypertensive agents:

a prospective placebo controlled study of sleep, mood state, and cognitive and sexual function in hypertensive males. Psychopharmacology 102: 163–170.

21. *True.* See Moore-Ede M C, Czeisler C A, Richardson G S 1983 Circadian timekeeping in health and disease. New England Journal of Medicine 309: 469–476.

22. *True.* See Woods J H, Katz J L, Winger G 1992 Benzodiazepines: use, abuse and consequences. Phamacological Revues 44: 151–347.

23. *True.* See Erlik Y, Tataryn I V, Meldrum D R, Lomax P, Bajorek J G, Judd H L 1981 Association of waking episodes with menopausal hot flushes. Journal of the American Medical Association 245: 1741–1744.

24. *False.* See Horne J A 1981 The effects of exercise upon sleep: a critical review. Biological Psychiatry 12: 241–290.

25. *False.* See Waters M A, Lee K A 1996 Differences between primigravidae and multigravidae mothers in sleep disturbances, fatigue, and functional status. Journal of Nurse Midwifery 41: 364–367.

26. *False.* Average sleep times are age-dependent. See Chapters 1 and 2.

27. *False.* Research shows that, when given to those unaccustomed to such fare, bedtime food drinks can actually disturb sleep. See Adam K 1980 Dietary habits and sleep after bedtime food drinks. Sleep 3: 47–58.

28. *False.* See Sadeh A, Dark I, Vohr B R 1996 Newborns' sleep–wake patterns: the role of maternal, delivery and infant factors. Early Human Development 44: 113–126.

29. *True.* See Kales A, Soldatos C R, Bixler E O et al 1980 Hereditary factors in sleepwalking and night terrors. British Journal of Psychiatry 137: 111–118.

30. *True.* See Ohayon M 1996 Epidemiologic study on insomnia in the general population. Sleep 19: S7–S15.

REFERENCES

American Psychiatric Association 1994 Diagnostic and statistical manual of mental disorders: DSM-IV. American Psychiatric Association, Washington DC

American Sleep Disorders Association 1990 The International Classification of Sleep Disorders: diagnostic and coding manual. American Sleep Disorders Association, Rochester, Minnesota

Anonymous 1991 Sleeping giant. (Editorial) Lancet 337: 1067

Aserinsky E, Kleitman N 1953 Regularly occurring periods of eye motility, and concomitant phenomena during sleep. Science 118: 273–274

Bliwise D 1993 Sleep in normal aging and dementia. Sleep 16: 40–81

Busby K A, Mercier L, Pivik R T 1994 Ontogenic variations in auditory arousal threshold during sleep. Psychophysiology 31: 182–188

Buysse D J, Reynolds C F, Kupfer D J et al 1994 Clinical diagnoses in 216 insomnia patients using the International Classification of Sleep Disorders (ICSD), DSM-IV and ICD-10 categories. A report from the APA/NIMH DSM-IV field trial. Sleep 17: 630–637

Dement W, Kleitman N 1957 The relation of eye movements during sleep to dream activity: an objective method for the study of dreaming. Journal of Experimental Psychology 53: 339–346

Karacan I, Williams R L, Thornby J I, Salis P J 1975 Sleep-related tumescence as a function of age. American Journal of Psychiatry 132: 932–937

McMahon R 1992 Nursing at night: a professional approach. Scutari Press, London

Nightingale F 1859 Notes on nursing. Reprinted 1952, Gerald Duckworth, London, pp 56–57

Rechtschaffen A, Kales A 1968 A manual of standardized terminology, techniques, and scoring system for sleep stages of human subjects. National Institute of Health Publication No 24, Government Printing Office, Washington DC

Thorpy M J 1994 Classification of sleep disorders. In: Kryger M H, Roth T, Dement W C (eds) Principles and practice of sleep medicine. W B Saunders, Philadelphia

World Health Organization 1993 The ICD-10 Classification of Mental and Behavioural Disorders. WHO, Geneva

Zepelin H, McDonald C S, Zammit G K 1984 Effects of age on auditory awakening thresholds. Journal of Gerontology 39(3): 294–300

The epidemiology of insomnia

Learning outcomes

This chapter examines the epidemiology and natural history of poor
sleep, and broadly addresses the question: who complains of insomnia?
On completing this chapter you should be able to:

- estimate the prevalence of insomnia in the general population
- describe age and gender trends in the prevalence of insomnia
- distinguish between the prevalence and the incidence of insomnia
- describe the most frequently reported psychological difference between
  good and poor sleepers.

INTRODUCTION

Epidemiology and nursing

Epidemiology is concerned with the occurrence and distribution
of illnesses and symptoms within populations. Using information
derived from population surveys or public records, epidemiological studies explore both the dimensions and dynamics of
health and ill-health. In addition to describing the overall levels
and course of particular disorders, epidemiology also provides
important insights into the origins and nature of those disorders,
and helps to identify those most at risk. Within the broader
context of medical research, this approach has proved invaluable
both in directing the attention of laboratory science, and in

monitoring the public impact of treatment programmes. Links between cigarette smoking and lung cancer, for example, were recognised by epidemiologists well before the aetiology of the disease was more fully understood.

From a nursing perspective, a working knowledge of the epidemiology of sleep disorders serves three important functions. First, epidemiology contributes (along with physiology, psychology, etc.) to a basic understanding of how sleep disorders appear, and how they operate in the real world. Second, such information helps to shape expectations in clinical practice (for example, by describing which patient groups are most at risk, and which symptoms are most frequently reported). And third, an improved epidemiological understanding can help to structure nursing management (by providing, for example, information on the probable duration of a complaint, and the likelihood of its recurrence). This chapter deals mainly with the descriptive epidemiology of insomnia, focusing in particular on *prevalence*, *incidence*, and *risk factors*. Because these terms are frequently misunderstood (or, in the case of incidence and prevalence, frequently confused), some basic epidemiological terms and concepts will first be considered.

Epidemiology: basic concepts

In epidemiological research, individuals with a particular illness, or who possess a particular health-related characteristic, are referred to as *cases*. Conversely, those who do not possess these characteristics can be referred to as non-cases. If a non-case is nevertheless eligible to become a case, the individual is said to be 'at-risk'. (Thus, children who have not yet had measles are 'at-risk' of becoming measles cases). *Prevalence* refers to the total number of existing cases at a given point in time, usually expressed as a proportion of the defined population. *Incidence*, on the other hand, refers to the number of new cases coming into existence over a defined period of time, expressed as a proportion of the total population at risk. Methodologically, these measurements are derived in quite different ways. Prevalence is usually estimated from cross-sectional studies where a defined population is screened at a particular point in time (yielding *point prevalence*). Incidence must be measured longitudinally, with those at risk monitored over a defined period (e.g. 1-year incidence; 5-year incidence, etc.). Values of incidence or prevalence which apply to the whole population are referred to as *overall* rates. However, because the incidence and/or prevalence of many disorders varies systematically with sex and age, incidence and prevalence rates are frequently reported separately by gender and age-group. Such rates are usually referred to as *age-specific* or *gender-specific* rates.

Both the differences, and the relationship between incidence and prevalence can usefully be illustrated by the analogy of the bathtub shown in Figure 2.1. Water running into the tub represents incidence (the new cases coming into existence). The total amount of water in the tub represents prevalence (the accumulation of existing cases), while the water leaving the tub represents recovery (or death). It follows, then, that since prevalence is a function of both incidence *and* recovery/death, it is not possible to predict incidence from prevalence alone. Some conditions may show a high incidence and a low prevalence, while others may show the reverse. Among children, for example, chickenpox has a fairly high incidence, but a fairly low prevalence (because recovery is rapid and cases do not accumulate). Conversely, baldness among men has a fairly low incidence, but a high prevalence (since recovery is rare and cases do, therefore, accumulate). In the study of insomnia, this point is quite important as we shall emphasise later in this chapter. *Risk factors* are those attributes which make it more likely that given individuals will become cases. Cigarette smoking, for example, is a risk factor for lung cancer, while obesity is a risk factor for coronary heart disease. Risk factors may be identified in (or inferred from) cross-sectional data, as correlates of the condition of interest. More usually, however, risk factor studies involve longitudinal follow-ups of non-cases (often incidence studies). It is through this type of longitudinal research that the typical course, or *natural history* of a disease or complaint is also evaluated.

INSOMNIA: PREVALENCE AND INCIDENCE

Prevalence

While formal diagnostic classification, of the type described in Chapter 1, is increasingly being used in epidemiological studies of insomnia (e.g. Foley et al 1995, Ford & Kamerow 1989) such

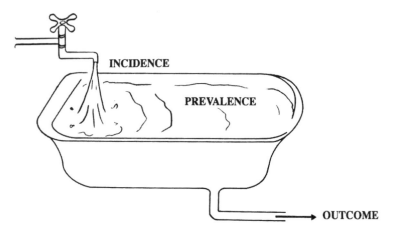

Figure 2.1 The concepts of incidence and prevalence are analogous to the water entering, and accumulating in this bathtub. Note that prevalence is a function of both incidence and outcome (recovery/death).

categorisation remains the exception. Nevertheless, since the seminal studies of McGhie & Russell (1962) in the UK, and Karacan et al (1976) in the USA, community surveys have been remarkably consistent in describing the prevalence and natural history of insomnia. Defined as subjectively reported dissatisfaction with sleep quantity or quality, insomnia affects approximately 10–15% of the adult population (see Partinen 1994 for review). Importantly, however, this overall prevalence estimate does not apply equally to all sections of the general population. In particular, prevalence varies according to age and gender, and is higher among lower income and lower educational attainment groups (Bixler et al 1979, Ford & Kamerow 1989, Habte-Gabr et al 1991, Karacan et al 1976, McGhie & Russell 1962).

There is considerable agreement that the prevalence of insomnia increases steadily with age (Bixler et al 1979, Gislason & Almqvist 1987, Jacquinet-Salord et al 1993, Karacan et al 1976, McGhie & Russell 1962, Mellinger et al 1985, Ohayon 1996), with estimates rising from approximately 5% among those aged 18–30 to over 30% among those aged 65 and over (Foley et al 1995, Gislason & Almqvist 1987, Mellinger et al 1985, Ohayon 1996; see Table 2.1). Epidemiological studies have also consistently shown that, across all ages, dissatisfaction with sleep is more common among women than among men (Foley et al 1995, Ford & Kamerow 1989, Ohayon

1996; see Fig. 2.2). It is interesting to note, however, that while epidemiological studies tend to show that women are more likely to report sleep difficulties, the electroencephalogram (EEG) studies indicate that it is men who tend to experience the greater fragmentation in their sleep architecture. The reasons for this discrepancy are not clearly understood, but possibly reflect cultural influences on the willingness of men and women to disclose symptoms and problems (see, for example Lindberg et al 1997, Rediehs et al 1990).

Increasing age is also associated with changes both in the nature, and the duration of sleep complaints. Problems in getting to sleep (sleep onset problems) tend to predominate among younger people, while problems staying asleep (sleep maintenance problems) become increasingly common in later life (Foley et al 1995, Gislason & Almqvist 1987; Fig. 2.3). Complaints of early morning awakening, also increase with age (Morgan 1996) but remain less common than sleep maintenance problems in elderly populations. Several epidemiological studies report data which indicate that symptoms of disturbed sleep are more *persistent* in later life (Hohagen et al 1994, Mellinger et al 1985). When asked to quantify the severity of insomnia, for example, older respondents are more likely than younger respondents to report that the problem occurs 'often or all the time' (Karacan et al 1976) or 'a lot' (Mellinger et al 1985).

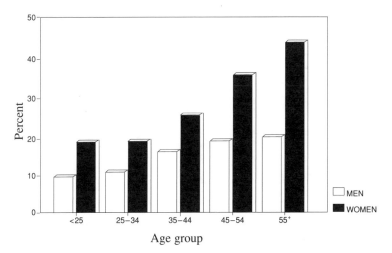

Figure 2.2 Typical relationship between age, gender, and the prevalence of insomnia (data summarised from Table 2.1).

Table 2.1 Age-specific and gender-specific prevalence rates of insomnia from community studies

Study	Gender	Overall	Age-specific (range in years)					
Karacan et al (1976)[a]	Women	15	9 (20–29)	15 (30–39)	16 (40–49)	17 (50–59)	23 (60–69)	29 (70+)
	Men	11	8 (20–29)	5 (30–39)	11 (40–49)	16 (50–59)	18 (60–69)	20 (70+)
Bixler et al (1979)[b]	Total*	32	23 (18–30)	37 (31–50)	40 (51+)			
Mellinger et al (1985)[c]	Total*	17	14 (18–34)	15 (35–49)		20 (50–64)	25 (65–79)	
Ford & Kamerow (1989)[d]	Women	12						
	Men	8						
	Total*		11 (18–25)	9 (26–44)	11 (45–64)	12 (65+)		
Jacquinet-Salord et al (1993)[e]	Women	26	15 (<25)	19 (25–34)	26 (35–44)	36 (45–54)	43 (55+)	
	Men	16	10 (<25)	12 (25–34)	17 (35–44)	19 (45–54)	23 (55+)	
Ohayon (1996)[f]	Women	24	15 (15–24)	16 (25–34)	22 (35–44)	26 (45–54)	30 (55–64)	37 (65+)
	Men	16	10 (15–24)	11 (25–34)	12 (35–44)	19 (45–54)	18 (55–64)	29 (65+)

*Combined figures for women/men only.

Insomnia defined as: [a]'trouble sleeping "often/all the time"; [b]current difficulty falling or staying asleep, or waking too early; [c]'had trouble and was bothered a lot' by 'trouble falling asleep or staying asleep'; [d]'had trouble falling asleep, staying asleep, or waking too early' for a period of 2 weeks or more, *and* consulted a professional about it, took medication for it, or stated that it interfered with life a lot, *and* 'if it was not always the result of physical illness'; [e]'self-perceived sleeping difficulties without sleeping tablets'; [f]unsatisfied with sleep *or* taking medication for sleep difficulties *or* (taking medication for) anxieties about sleep difficulties.

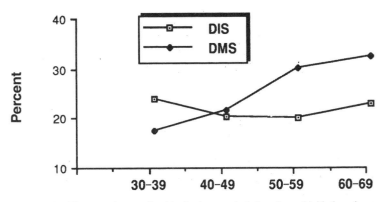

Figure 2.3 The prevalence of subjectively reported disorders of initiating sleep (DIS or problems getting to sleep) and disorders of maintaining sleep (DMS or problems staying asleep) among men (source: data from Gislason & Almqvist 1987).

It was pointed out above that if a proportion of new cases fail to recover (i.e. if they become chronic) then, over time, cases will tend to accumulate. (This, of course, applies only to non-fatal conditions.) Since insomnia can become chronic at any age, and since it is not in itself a fatal condition, it follows that cases will tend to accumulate in older age groups. Thus, for example, some 30-year-olds who develop chronic insomnia may, 10 years later, appear as 40-year-olds with insomnia, and so on. Given this, it is important to recognise that the high prevalence of insomnia *in* old age is not necessarily due *to* old age. Rather, the sleep problems reported by many of those in their 50s and 60s may have originated much earlier in life. In a representative sample of adults aged 18–66+, Bixler et al (1979) found that the average age of insomnia onset was 38 years. Similarly, from sleep histories collected in face-to-face interviews, Morgan (1989) found that up to 78% of elderly chronic insomniacs develop their sleep problems before (and sometimes well before) the age of 65 (Fig. 2.4).

Insomnia and hypnotic drug use

While community surveys provide direct evidence of prevalence, levels of insomnia can also be estimated indirectly from patterns of hypnotic drug use. Like subjective complaints of poor sleep, hypnotic drug use also increases steadily with age and, at all ages,

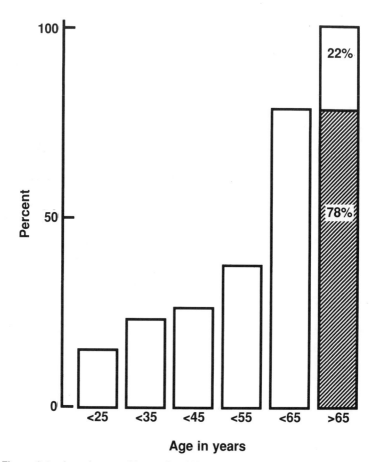

Figure 2.4   Age of onset of insomnia within a random sample of poor sleepers aged 65–74 (source: Morgan 1989).

tends to be greater among women (e.g. Jacquinet-Salord et al 1993; Fig. 2.5). It is important to recognise, however, that patterns of hypnotic drug use, and patterns of reported insomnia differ in at least two important ways. First, complaints of poor sleep are much more prevalent than hypnotic drug use (e.g. Jacquinet-Salord et al 1993), suggesting, perhaps, that many people manage their own sleep problems. And second, differences between men and women appear to be greater for hypnotic drug use than for subjectively reported insomnia, suggesting either gender differences in medical consultation levels, or perhaps a gender bias in prescribing.

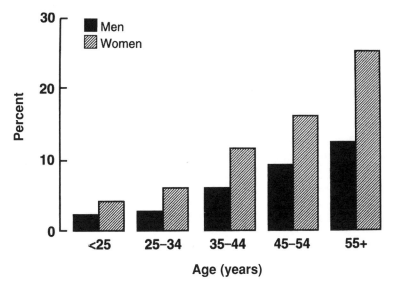

Figure 2.5   Prevalence of hypnotic drug use within a wage-earning sample (data from Jacquinet-Salord et al 1993).

Overall, then, while hypnotic drug prescribing levels provide a useful proxy for the underlying sleep complaint, they generally underestimate true levels of insomnia.

Incidence

In contrast to the abundance of prevalence data, information on the incidence of insomnia (i.e. the rate at which new cases come into existence) is scarce. Nevertheless, in one of the few studies to examine this issue, a clear, though modest, age gradient in the 1-year incidence of insomnia was present, with incident complaints rising from 5.7% among those aged 18–25, to 7.3% among those aged 65 and over (Ford & Kamerow 1989). Lower estimates of incidence for the age group 65 years and over are reported by Morgan & Clarke (1997), who nevertheless found that incidence continued to show a clear age gradient after 65 years. For each year at risk in a 4-year follow-up, these researchers found incidence rates of 2.8%, 3.2% and 3.5% for the age groups 65–69, 70–74 and 75–79 respectively.

INSOMNIA AND RISK FACTORS

From the information reviewed so far, it is reasonable to conclude that both increased age, and female gender, may be viewed as risk factors for insomnia. The experimental and epidemiological evidence also points to the existence of psychological and health factors which are strongly associated with the onset and/or the maintenance of disturbed sleep. Many of these factors will be discussed in more detail in subsequent chapters. Here, mention will be made of two factors which, broadly, are associated with an increased risk of insomnia: anxiety-related personality characteristics, and health status.

Anxiety-related personality characteristics

Psychologists distinguish between two types of anxiety. State anxiety refers to those feelings of fear or nervousness experienced in response to a particular event or situation. The quite normal tension experienced before an interview or examination provides an example of state anxiety. Trait anxiety, on the other hand, refers to the level of anxiety which typifies an individual's behaviour. If, for example, we describe someone as being an anxious sort of person, we are using the construct of trait anxiety. It follows from this that while state anxiety is labile, trait anxiety is a relatively enduring personal characteristic.

Studies comparing the personality profiles of otherwise healthy good and poor sleepers have found consistent differences among young (Monroe 1967), middle-aged (Adam et al 1986) and elderly (Morgan et al 1989) subjects. In all cases, poor sleepers have shown significantly elevated levels of state and/or trait anxiety (Fig. 2.6). Similar relationships between insomnia and anxiety have also been found in sleep clinic patients (Kales et al 1983) and representative population samples (Hyyppa et al 1991).

It is possible that such characteristics may act as risk factors for insomnia either directly, by contributing to levels of emotional arousal antagonistic to sleep (Kales et al 1983), or indirectly by lowering the threshold at which sleep is perceived to be a problem. Just as medicine uses the construct of 'pain thresholds' to explain why some patients report greater discomfort than others, these personality characteristics may be considered as markers for those whose sleep is inherently more vulnerable, and whose threshold for reporting dissatisfaction is consequently lower.

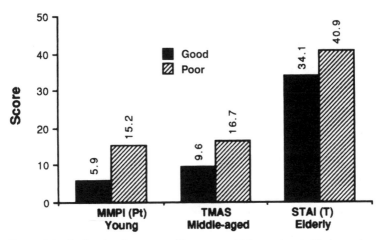

Figure 2.6   Anxiety levels compared in young, middle-aged and elderly good and poor sleepers. Measurements are: MMPI (Minnesota Multiphasic Personality Inventory – psychasthenia scale); TMAS (Taylor Manifest Anxiety Scale); STAI (Spielberger State–Trait Anxiety Inventory – trait scale). (Data from: Adam et al 1986, Monroe 1967, Morgan 1989.)

Health status

As a correlate of psychological well-being, insomnia continues to be regarded as a useful indicant of mental ill-health, appearing as a prominent diagnostic feature in both the ICD-10 (World Health Organization 1993), and DSM-IV (American Psychiatric Association 1994) classifications of depression. In addition, insomnia is also clearly related to physical ill-health, emerging as a concomitant of pain, discomfort and the (state) anxieties of ill-health (see Closs 1992a,b). Assuming a 'pie' model of causes underlying insomnia, where each 'slice' represents a causal factor, the *relative* contribution of mental and physical ill health to levels of insomnia has been assessed in a number of epidemiological studies. The extent to which psychiatric problems are associated with insomnia in the general population, for example, was explored by Ford & Kamerow (1989). In this survey of nearly 8000 adult respondents of all ages, it was found that approximately 40% of all insomnias were associated with some form of psychological disturbance (Fig. 2.7A). Reviewing the literature for older respondents, Morgan (1996) found slightly higher levels of insomnia-related psychological disturbance (Fig. 2.7B). Of course, psychological and somatic factors are not always clearly distinct in clinical practice, where physical ill-health and emotional disturbance frequently coexist (e.g. Schramm et al 1994). Nevertheless, these studies do reinforce the important general point that, in nursing and medicine, insomnias frequently cut across the boundaries of clinical specialities.

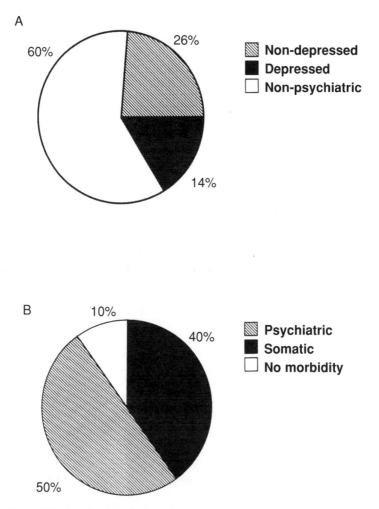

Figure 2.7 Levels of psychological/somatic disorder associated with insomnia in community samples: (A) of all ages; and (B) of older people.

CONSEQUENCES OF INSOMNIA

The impact of insomnia on morale and health has long been recognised, with early clinical accounts showing an eloquence (and an attention to detail) rare in today's research literature. In a lecture reported in *The Lancet* in 1832, Dr George Sigmond (a pharmacologist at the Windmill Street School of Medicine, London) told his students that: 'Obstinate sleeplessness is a malady that preys upon every system, disordering every function; during the darkness, the silence, and the solitude of night, all the causes of conflicting passion, of anxiety, and of corroding feeling, rise up with redoubled energy, and haunt the broken spirit.'

In the late 20th century, insomnia remains a major cause of personal distress. However, in addition to quantifying the levels of such distress, epidemiology can also assess the public health impact of disordered sleep.

Insomnia is both widely reported and widely treated in general practice, where hypnotic drugs remain the treatment of choice (Hohagen et al 1994, Jacquinet-Salord et al 1993, Pharoah & Melzer 1995, Weyerer & Dilling 1991). In England, for example, the total volume of general practice prescriptions for hypnotics shows only a modest decline from 13.6 million in 1980 to 12.0 million in 1992, the last year for which published data are available (Department of Health 1982–1992; Fig. 2.8). During the same period, prescriptions for sedatives and tranquillisers fell from 18.9 million to 8.6 million. Similar trends have been reported for Scotland (Common Services Agency for the Scottish Health Service 1980–1992), Wales (Welsh Office 1983–1992) and elsewhere in Europe (Ekedahl et al 1993). While hypnotics have long been associated with unwanted side-effects, particularly residual sedation on the day following drug use (see Ch. 10), the research evidence increasingly suggests that untreated insomnia can also significantly impair daytime functioning. Thus, in epidemiological studies, both the principal symptom associated with insomnia (daytime sleepiness) and hypnotic drug consumption have been independently associated with reduced work performance (Leger 1994), absenteeism (Jacquinet-Salord et al 1993, Leger 1994), and road traffic accidents (Ray et al 1992, Jacquinet-Salord et al 1993, Leger 1994) in the general population. Among elderly people, sleepiness (Leger 1995) and hypnotic drug use (Ray et al 1987, Wysowski et al 1996) have also been specifically implicated as causes of falls and fractured neck of femur. Clearly, then, the epidemiological evidence emphasises the need not only to treat insomnia, but also the need to treat insomnia appropriately.

CONCLUSIONS

Defined as subjectively reported dissatisfaction with sleep quantity or quality, insomnia represents a major public health issue affecting up to 10–15% of the adult population. Insofar as they are associated with an increased likelihood of reporting poor quality sleep, older age and female gender may be regarded as risk factors for insomnia. In addition, some individuals seem constitutionally predisposed to insomnia, through anxiety-related personality characteristics. It follows, therefore, that in clinical situations, circumstances and experiences which can disturb sleep are often superimposed upon existing susceptibilities. These additional factors will be considered in the next chapter.

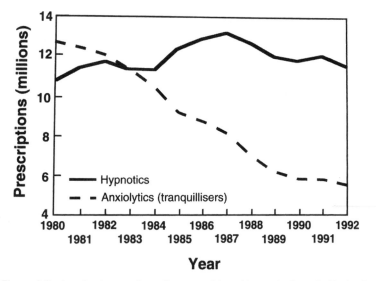

Figure 2.8 Levels of general practice prescribing of hypnotic drugs in England: 1982–1992 (source: Health and Personal Social Service Statistics for England 1982–1993). After 1992 new, more conservative, definitions of 'hypnotic' were introduced by the Department of Health in England. A total of 8.4 million prescriptions, defined according to these new criteria, were issued in 1996 (source: personal communication from the Department of Health).

REFERENCES

Adam K, Tomeny M, Oswald I 1986 Physiological and psychological differences between good and poor sleepers. Journal of Psychiatric Research 20(4): 301–316

American Psychiatric Association 1994 Diagnostic and statistical manual of mental disorders: DSM-IV. American Psychiatric Association, Washington DC

Bixler E O, Kales A, Soldatos C R, Kales J D, Healey S 1979 Prevalence of sleep disorders in the Los Angeles metropolitan area. American Journal of Psychiatry 136: 1257–1262

Closs S J 1992a Post-operative patients' views of sleep, pain and recovery. Journal of Clinical Nursing 1: 83–88

Closs S J 1992b Patients' night-time pain, analgesic provision and sleep after surgery. International Journal of Nursing Studies 29(4): 381–392

Department of Health 1982–1992 Health and Personal Social Service Statistics for England. HMSO, London

Common Services Agency for the Scottish Health Service 1980–1992 Scottish Health Statistics. CSASHS, Edinburgh

Ekedahl A, Lidbeck J, Lithman T, Noreen D, Melander A 1993 Benzodiazepine prescribing patterns in a high-prescribing Scandinavian community. European Journal of Clinical Pharmacology 44: 141–146

Foley D J, Monjan A A, Brown S L, Simonsick E M, Wallace R B, Blazer D G 1995 Sleep complaints among elderly persons: an epidemiologic study of three communities. Sleep 18: 425–432

Ford D E, Kamerow D B 1989 Epidemiologic study of sleep disturbances and psychiatric disorders. Journal of the American Medical Association 262: 1479–1484

Gislason T, Almqvist M 1987 Somatic diseases and sleep complaints. Acta Medica Scandinavica 221: 475–481

Habte-Gabr E, Wallace R B, Colsher P L, Hulbert J R, White L R, Smith I M 1991 Sleep patterns in rural elders: demographic, health, and psychobehavioral correlates. Journal of Clinical Epidemiology 44: 5–13

Hohagen F, Käppler C, Schramm E, Rink K, Weyerer S, Riemann D, Berger M 1994 Prevalence of insomnia in general practice attenders and the current treatment modalities. Acta Psychiatrica Scandinavica 90: 102–108

Hyyppa M T, Kronholm E, Mattlar C E 1991 Mental well-being of good sleepers in a random population sample. British Journal of Medical Psychology 64: 25–34

Jacquinet-Salord M C, Lang T, Fouriaud C, Nicoulet I, Bingham A 1993 Sleeping tablet consumption, self reported quality of sleep, and working conditions. Journal of Epidemiology and Community Health 47: 64–68

Kales A, Caldwell A B, Soldatos C R, Bixler E O, Kales J D 1983 Biopsychobehavioral correlates of insomnia II: pattern specificity and consistency with MMPI. Psychosomatic Medicine 45: 341–356

Karacan I, Thornby J I, Anch H et al 1976 The prevalence of sleep disturbance in a primarily urban Florida county. Social Science and Medicine 10: 239–244

Leger D 1994 The cost of sleep related road accidents. Sleep 17, 84–93

Leger D 1995 The cost of sleepiness: a response to comments. Sleep 18: 281–284

Lindberg E, Janson C, Gislason T, Bjornsson E, Hetta J, Boman G 1997 Sleep disturbances in a young adult population: can gender differences be explained by differences in psychological status? Sleep 20: 381–387

McGhie A, Russell S M 1962 The subjective assessment of normal sleep patterns. Journal of Mental Science 108: 642–654

Mellinger G D, Balter M B, Uhlenhuth E H 1985 Insomnia and its treatment. Archives of General Psychiatry 42: 225–232

Monroe L J 1967 Psychological and physiological differences between good and poor sleepers. Journal of Abnormal Psychology 72: 255–264

Morgan K 1989 Why do old people complain of poor sleep? In: Horne J A, Page M L (eds) Sleep disorders: current approaches. Duphar Medical Relations, Southampton, pp 11–19

Morgan K 1996 Mental health factors in late-life insomnia. Reviews in Clinical Gerontology 6: 75–83

Morgan K, Clarke D 1997 Longitudinal trends in late-life insomnia: implications for prescribing. Age and Ageing 26: 179–184

Morgan K, Healey D W, Healey P J 1989 Factors influencing persistent subjective insomnia in old age: a follow-up study of good and poor sleepers aged 65–74. Age and Ageing 18: 117–122

Ohayon M 1996 Epidemiologic-study on insomnia in the general-population. Sleep 19: S7–S15

Partininen M 1994 Epidemiology of sleep disorders. In: Roth T, Dement W C (eds) Principles and practice of sleep medicine. Saunders, Philadelphia, pp 437–452

Pharoah P D P, Melzer D 1995 Variations in prescribing of hypnotics, anxiolytics and antidepressants between 61 general practices. British Journal of General Practice 45: 595–599

Ray W A et al 1987 Psychotropic drug use and the risk of hip fracture. New England Journal of Medicine 316: 363–369

Rediehs M H, Reis J S, Creason N S 1990 Sleep in old age: focus on gender differences. Sleep 13: 410–424

Schramm E, Hohagen F, Kappler C, Grasshoff U, Berger M 1994 Mental comorbidity of chronic insomnia in general practice attenders using DSM-III-R. Acta Psychiatrica Scandinavica 91: 10–17

Welsh Office 1983–1992. Health and Personal Social Service Statistics for Wales, Cardiff

Weyerer S, Dilling H 1991 Prevalence and treatment of insomnia in the community – results from the upper Bavarian field-study. Sleep 14: 392–398

World Health Organization 1993 The ICD-10 Classification of Mental and Behavioural Disorders. WHO, Geneva

Wysowski D K, Baum C, Ferguson W J, Lundin F, Ng M J, Hammerstrom T 1996 Sedative-hypnotic drugs and the risk of hip fracture. Journal of Clinical Epidemiology 49: 111–113

3

Causes and correlates of disturbed sleep

Learning outcomes

This chapter considers some of the events, circumstances and clinical conditions which can reduce sleep quality. On completing this chapter you should be able to:

- name three social drugs which interfere with normal sleep
- define the diagnostic criteria for sleep apnoea
- describe the changes in sleep structure caused by anxiety
- describe the symptoms of sleep terrors in children.

INTRODUCTION

As suggested in the previous chapter, a variety of circumstances, conditions and personal susceptibilities contribute to the overall prevalence of insomnia reported in community studies. Some of these factors are external to the sleeper; some are associated with waking behaviour; some are associated with physical or psychological problems; and others represent specific disorders of sleep mechanisms (see Box 3.1). This chapter considers the nature and the effects of some of the more common, or the more disruptive causes of disturbed sleep. Since the aim is to provide an overview of sleep disturbances relevant to nursing practice, the review is selective, and necessarily brief. It is intended, nevertheless, that the issues described here will support the more general point that, while a variety of circumstances can influence sleep quality, many of these circumstances can be controlled, and their impact modified.

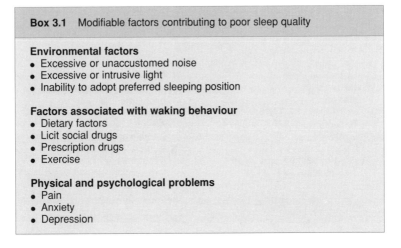

Box 3.1 Modifiable factors contributing to poor sleep quality

Environmental factors
- Excessive or unaccustomed noise
- Excessive or intrusive light
- Inability to adopt preferred sleeping position

Factors associated with waking behaviour
- Dietary factors
- Licit social drugs
- Prescription drugs
- Exercise

Physical and psychological problems
- Pain
- Anxiety
- Depression

EXTERNAL CAUSES OF SLEEP DISTURBANCE

Some causes of sleep disruption are due to the environment, which may be noisy, too hot, cold or light, or not conducive to lying in one's preferred sleeping position. Evidence linking these factors to sleep quality is presented below.

Noise

Noise is a major cause of sleep disturbance, in many different situations. It disturbs normal sleep stage progression and increases frequency of awakening. Noise can increase the number of body movements during the night, as well as the frequency of stage shifts and awakening. Fortunately for most people, adaptation to sleeping in a noisy environment occurs rapidly (within a few days), but for most, this adaptation is never complete. Noise which has disturbed sleep is not always remembered the following morning, and as a result may manifest itself as daytime sleepiness rather than a complaint of insomnia.

Different individuals have different tolerance levels when it comes to noise. Some remain oblivious throughout thunderstorms and neighbours' wild parties, while others are disturbed by the slightest creak of a floorboard. Women appear to be more sensitive to noise than men (Nivison & Endresen 1993) and older people are more sensitive than younger ones (Zepelin et al 1984). The latter found a significant decline in the intensity of noise required to arouse people from sleep with increasing age, and this reduction was present in all sleep stages but greatest in stage 4. In this increasingly noisy urban society, night-time noise is increasingly a problem for light sleepers. The significance, rather than the volume of noise is also important. A mother may sleep through a violent thunderstorm, while waking at the smallest whimper produced by her child.

Outside the home, traffic, aeroplanes and noisy neighbours may all produce unacceptable levels of noise. While constant noise is relatively easy to adjust to, it is sudden or intermittent noises which tend to be the most disruptive. Car alarms are a relatively recent intrusion into night-time peace and quiet. Loud music is frequently a cause for complaint, where the bass thumping is transmitted throughout buildings. A study of environmental noise in Valencia showed that the major sources of noise which disturbed sleep were traffic, neighbours and factories. About one-tenth of those interviewed had moved bedroom or slept with windows closed as a result (Aparicio et al 1993). A review of the effects of traffic noise on sleep showed that there is not yet a consensus view on habituation to noise (Kawada 1995). However, it does seem that overnight rapid eye movement (REM) sleep decreases with exposure to noise, and there is a linear relationship between noise levels and the rate of sleep stage shifts or waking. Another, more recent review of the effects of aircraft noise on sleep confirmed that it can cause changes in the sleeping electroencephalogram (EEG), including more wakefulness and difficulty in maintaining sleep (Morrell et al 1997). Those with a pre-existing psychological or psychiatric condition were more susceptible to the effects of noise.

Normal family life can involve babies crying during the night, children sneaking into their parents' bed, or a snoring partner. Disturbances due to children are usually short-term and can be minimised by good parenting skills. Health visitors may have an important role to play in helping parents with such problems.

Snoring is often a source of disturbance as much for the partners as for the snorers themselves. While snorers are usually unaware of the noise they are making, those sharing the bed may have their sleep severely disrupted by it. Snoring is caused by air turbulence in the pharynx, usually due to nasal blockage or soft tissues obstructing the air flow. Recent survey evidence shows that snoring affects approximately 40% of the UK population, and is most prevalent among men, cigarette smokers, the obese, and those who consume large amounts of coffee (≥ 6 cups per day; Ohayon et al 1997).

Encouraging the obese snorer to lose weight is the first step. Discouraging the snorer from lying on his or her back can sometimes reduce the obstruction. There are several devices available which dilate the nostrils during sleep and these may succeed in stopping snoring. As a last resort, surgery to remove the obstructing tissues may be undertaken. Snoring may also be symptomatic of sleep apnoea, which is discussed later on.

Domestic noise may be coped with by using ear plugs. These vary in construction and comfort; some are pre-shaped, albeit soft in texture, while others are made of malleable wax, which can be moulded to fit individual ears. These can reduce disturbances to sleep due to noise. However, not everyone finds them comfortable, and there is also the problem of not hearing the alarm clock go off in the morning.

Temperature

As they do with noise, individuals vary markedly in their sensitivity to temperature. Both ambient temperature and body temperature have been shown to influence the normal sleep–wake cycle. Muzet et al (1984) found that 'even slight changes of the ambient temperature within the thermoneutral zone can induce modifications of sleep structure'. Unclothed and uncovered subjects in a room temperature of 26°C and below have been shown to wake up because of feeling cold (Kendel & Schmidt-Kessen 1973).

Interestingly, deviations from optimal temperatures do not appear to inhibit falling asleep, rather they disrupt sleep maintenance. Wakefulness and stage 1 increase and REM decreases. The changes in the structure of sleep are similar for heat and cold, but cold tends to produce more pronounced effects. Bedroom (or ward) temperature should be kept at a comfortable level, and more or less bedclothes used as required.

Fever has been found to be associated with a greater number of awakenings, increased total waking time and reduced amounts of slow wave sleep (SWS) and REM. Elevated ambient temperature produces similar results (Karacan et al 1978, Otto 1973). The duration of the REM phase is shortened in artificially induced fever (Karacan et al 1968) as well as at high ambient temperature. The duration of REM sleep is negatively correlated with body temperature and body temperature influences sleep duration (Zulley 1980; Zulley & Schultz 1980). These findings suggest that active management of pyrexial patients, perhaps by giving antipyretic drugs such as aspirin (or paracetamol for children), might improve their sleep.

Light

Again, individual sensitivity to light is variable. There is little doubt, however, that strong light is a powerful zeitgeber, providing a major stimulus for the body to function in its daytime mode. It is thought to do this by inhibiting the secretion of the hormone melatonin from the pineal gland (Short 1993). Melatonin acts on the 'circadian clock' situated in the suprachiasmatic nuclei of the hypothalamus. It tells the brain that it is night-time, and therefore time to sleep. Maintaining cues of light and darkness can help to synchronise circadian rhythms, including sleep. It is therefore important that, for example, patients in intensive care units are not exposed to constant bright light. Similarly, night-shift workers are likely to sleep better in a dark environment during the day. Lesser lights at night may act merely as distractions, such as flashing lights in hospital wards, or inappropriately positioned night-lights. Even though dim, these may be directly in the line of sight of patients, making it more difficult for them to sleep.

Sleep position

Most of us sleep lying down. There are occasions, however, when we are obliged to sleep in unaccustomed positions, such as when we are travelling long distances in cars or aeroplanes. A study of the effect of the angle at which the back was inclined during sleep showed that it was associated with poorer sleep than when lying flat. Total sleep time was reduced and there was greater wakefulness compared with usual sleep in bed (Nicholson & Stone 1987). This kind of insomnia is unpleasant, but is easily remedied by subsequent sleep under normal conditions.

WAKING BEHAVIOUR AND SLEEP DISTURBANCE

What we eat, which drugs we ingest (on prescription or socially) and the exercise we take may all, directly or indirectly, influence how well we sleep.

Diet

There has been considerable research into the effects of diet on sleep but few clear findings have emerged. The roles of particular nutrients are not clear, but the effects of dieting (weight reduction) itself are more convincing. While acute fasting is related to an increase in the amount of SWS, prolonged starvation increases the rate of protein catabolism and time spent awake, and SWS and REM are both reduced. Weight loss, such as that produced by anorexia nervosa, is associated with changes in sleep. Total sleep time is reduced, together with more broken sleep and earlier waking (Crisp & Stonehill 1973). Conversely, as might be expected, weight gain is associated with longer total sleeping time, later waking and less broken sleep. There appear to be correlations between percentage of ideal body weight and the duration of sleep, especially SWS and total sleep time (TST) (Levy et al 1987, 1988).

The biochemical effects of diet on sleep are not all clear, but since departure from dietary habit appears to disturb sleep, eating habits and preferences should, as far as is possible, be maintained in the home and the hospital. (This principal forms part of the 'sleep hygiene' practices described in Ch. 6.) The possibility that certain foods actually promote sleep has, however, been investigated. Brezinova & Oswald (1972) found that Horlicks apparently enhanced sleep by increasing its total duration and reducing periods of wakefulness. Unfortunately, the volunteers who had participated in the study were a self-selected group of people who may have preferred milky night-time drinks anyway. Subsequent research by Adam (1980) found that among those accustomed to foods taken late at night, Horlicks significantly improved sleep duration and continuity (relative to non-drink nights). However, among those unaccustomed to late night food, Horlicks at bedtime was associated with shorter, more broken sleep. The maintenance of dietary *habit*, therefore, emerges as the important factor here. It should also be remembered that many traditional milky beverages such as hot chocolate and coffee contain caffeine, which can seriously interfere with sleep (see below).

Social drugs

Alcohol, nicotine and caffeine are socially acceptable drugs which may produce marked effects on sleep. Illegal drugs such as amphetamines, cocaine and opioids also affect sleep. Many people use alcohol to relax themselves if they are physically tense. Nevertheless, alcohol is not a good hypnotic drug. It accelerates sleep onset and reduces wakefulness for the first 3–4 hours of the night, but it disturbs sleep patterns later on in the night, suppressing REM and producing frequent awakenings and non-restorative sleep. Some of this is due to physical discomfort such as headache and stomach irritation, and large amounts usually cause awakenings in the early hours owing to a full bladder. Withdrawal from regular alcohol intake (similarly to hypnotic drugs), will result in disturbed sleep.

Caffeine is a much more potent central nervous system (CNS) stimulant than is generally realised, although individuals have different sensitivities to its effects. In doses of 1 g, for example, caffeine can produce insomnia, cardiac arrhythmias and delirium, while the ingestion of more than 5 g can be fatal. An average cup of instant coffee contains about 85–100 mg of caffeine, while strong ground coffee can contain up to 200 mg. The effects of caffeine are prolonged in children and pregnant women, and may be toxic at lower doses for these groups. It has been shown that as little as two cups of a caffeinated drink before bedtime can disturb the sleeping EEG (Karacan et al 1976). Ingested in coffee, caffeine levels in blood peak after about 1 hour, with an elimination half-life of about 3–7 hours. Consequently, caffeine taken in the early to mid evening is still likely to interfere with sleep onset. If it is taken directly before bed, it is more likely to cause waking later in the night (see Fig. 3.1). Stopping caffeine ingestion can improve sleep, and has been shown to reduce the number of night-time awakenings and requests for hypnotics among psychiatric inpatients (Edelstein et al 1984). However, abrupt withdrawal by those whose intake exceeds 400–500 mg per day can produce unpleasant withdrawal symptoms, such as headache, irritability and fatigue. Gradual withdrawal can minimise these problems.

It is not only coffee which contains caffeine, but also tea (including some herbal teas), hot chocolate, cola and other soft drinks such as Mountain Dew and Dr Pepper. Caffeine is also found in some over-the-counter medicines, such as Aqua-Ban

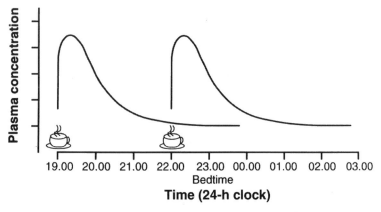

Figure 3.1 Plasma caffeine levels following coffee ingestion. Coffee ingestion at 19.00 will result in significant caffeine levels at bedtime (23.00). Coffee ingestion near bedtime will produce caffeine levels active for much of the sleep period.

diuretic and Sudafed decongestant. It is also an ingredient of several mild oral analgesics. A recent study of the effects of 'occult caffeine', that is caffeine hidden in such medications, showed it to be a significant cause of difficulty in getting to sleep amongst older people (Brown et al 1995).

Nicotine is another CNS stimulant which is associated with difficulty in falling asleep (Soldatos et al 1980), although its direct effects on sleep are poorly understood. Among heavy smokers, nicotine *withdrawal*, on the other hand, has also been associated with disturbed sleep, particularly increases in sleep fragmentation (Prosise et al 1994). Interestingly, such withdrawal effects may be avoided by the use of 'patches' providing transdermal nicotine (Wolter et al 1996).

Illegal stimulants such as cocaine and methamphetamine reduce sleepiness and suppress sleep itself. Acute use of such drugs can result in the users going for days without sleep, and then taking excessive sleep once the bout is over. Chronic use of stimulants at low to moderate doses can produce tolerance to the sleep-reducing effects. Withdrawal from such drugs is associated with an increased TST and REM, followed by a period of insomnia for around 2 weeks. SWS often takes longer to recover, remaining low for several weeks. The acute use of opioids such as heroin reduces sleep efficiency, TST, SWS and REM. With chronic use (more than 1 week) tolerance to the effects develops.

Prescription drugs

Drugs which act on the CNS can have profound effects on sleep. CNS depressants include not only hypnotics (discussed in Ch. 10), sedatives and tranquillisers, but also anticonvulsants, antihypertensives, antidepressants, antihistamines and beta-blockers. An overview of common drugs which can interfere with sleep is shown in Box 3.2. All of these may produce daytime sleepiness, and some (for example beta-blockers) can disturb nocturnal sleep (see Kostis et al 1990). The somewhat paradoxical impact of hypnotic drugs on sleep is explained in Chapter 10. CNS stimulants include amphetamines, sympathomimetic drugs, and analeptics. These can delay the onset of sleep and reduce total sleeping time, and can produce daytime symptoms of anxiety, irritability and difficulty in concentrating. Other drugs may have similar effects in a dose-dependent manner, including oncological chemotherapeutic agents and thyroid preparations.

Box 3.1 Prescription drugs which may contribute to insomnia (Reite et al 1997, Roehrs et al 1994)

- Beta-blockers
- Corticosteroids
- Monoamine oxidase inhibitors
- Calcium blockers
- Thyroxine
- Thiazides
- Methyldopa
- Antimetabolites
- Bronchodilators
- Benzodiazepine hypnotics (see Ch. 10)
- CNS stimulants (e.g. amphetamine)

Exercise

It is conventional wisdom that daytime exercise makes us sleep better during the night. However, although much research evidence supports this idea (e.g. Hauri 1992, Vuori et al 1988), some does not (e.g. Trinder et al 1988). There seems to be a difference in the importance of exercise, depending on whether the individuals concerned are good or poor sleepers to begin with. A recent meta-analysis examined 38 studies into the effects of exercise on good sleepers (Youngstedt et al 1997), and concluded that exercise had different effects on different aspects of sleep. Overall, it extended TST, and in particular stage 2 sleep. REM sleep was reduced. Outcomes for SWS were variable; it decreased significantly in almost as many studies as it was found to increase in. However, the magnitude of these changes was slight, ranging from 10 minutes for SWS to a mere 1.7 minutes for stage 2 sleep. Exercise does not, therefore, appear to have quite the profound effects sometimes claimed for it.

Research into the effects of exercise on poor sleepers is, perhaps, more interesting. For example, a randomised controlled trial designed to test the hypothesis that exercise would improve both the quality of sleep and daytime activity levels in depressed elderly people was reported recently (Singh et al 1997). They found that exercise was significantly more successful in the poor sleepers than the good ones – this may be because of the indirect effect on sleep, via a reduction in depression.

PHYSICAL AND PSYCHOLOGICAL PROBLEMS

Pain

Sufferers of both acute and chronic pain are likely to report some degree of sleep disturbance (see Haythornthwaite et al 1991). The population of chronic pain sufferers in the UK is estimated to be around 5 million people (Diamond 1991), a figure which includes a high proportion of elderly people, and the more frail. For example, one-third of a group of nursing home residents cited pain as a major cause of sleep disturbance (Gentili et al 1997). Sources of chronic pain are varied, including conditions such as rheumatoid arthritis, low back pain, fibromyalgia syndrome and the burning foot pain of diabetic neuropathy.

A study of pain clinic patients showed that those who were poor sleepers were less active, more anxious and depressed and in more severe pain than good sleepers (Pilowsky et al 1985). For many it is the pain itself which disturbs sleep directly, while pain may also have an indirect effect in sleep, through the psychological responses to pain such as depression (Phillips & Cousins 1986). Furthermore, some disease processes themselves can cause sleep pathology. For example, active rheumatoid arthritis releases cytokines which modulate sleep (Kreuger & Majde 1995).

Some kinds of chronic pain have shown a circadian rhythm, often worsening during the night (Glyn et al 1976). For example, dyspepsia and ulcer pain are frequently worse during the night.

Chronic back pain sufferers also exhibit circadian variations in pain intensity; for some it is worse during the day and for others worse during the night; and the majority of sciatic pain sufferers experience most severe pain during the evening and at night (Domzal et al 1983). Some kinds of acute pain also exhibit circadian patterns. For example, the onset of chest pain due to angina has a bimodal frequency, most attacks occurring between 23.30 and 03.00 and between 06.30 and 08.30 (Thompson et al 1991). Cluster headaches are precipitated during REM sleep.

A study monitoring the effects of both cutaneous and deep pain on sleep produced complex results (Drewes et al 1997). They found that muscle pain caused waking and a decrease in SWS; joint pain produced widespread changes throughout the whole EEG, particularly a reduction in the lowest frequencies; and cutaneous stimulation produced some changes, but these were poorly defined. Currently, the direct effects of different kinds of pain on sleep patterns are poorly understood.

Anxiety

A large study of almost 8000 people showed that insomnia was related strongly to major anxiety and depression disorders (Ford & Kamerow 1989). Sufferers of chronic tension-anxiety are habitually tense, restless and insomniac. It has been suggested that anxious, perfectionist personalities tend to internalise stressful life events, producing heightened emotional and physiological arousal. Those suffering from a generalised anxiety disorder often report that they find it difficult to relax and stop worrying when it is time to go to bed. Physiologically, anxiety produces an increase of plasma noradrenaline levels owing to increased activity of the sympathetic nervous system, and thus exacerbating symptoms of insomnia. The sleep changes associated with anxiety can be prolonged and severe. They include difficulty in initiating and maintaining sleep, and an increased time awake during the night compared with normal sleepers (Akiskal et al 1984, Sitaram et al 1984). A complementary study comparing anxious and depressed outpatients showed that anxiety sufferers had greater sleep latencies, more time awake and reduced SWS (Reynolds et al 1983).

Overall, then, those suffering from generalised anxiety disorders tend to report that the quality of their sleep is poor, together with difficulty in falling asleep and restless, broken sleep. Nurses have a role in helping patients to identify the causes of their anxiety, and in some cases may be able to make practical suggestions for dealing with them. They should also be able to recognise when anxiety (or tension) may benefit from a more formal therapeutic approach (see Chapter 8).

Depression

Frequently accompanied by symptoms of anxiety, depression can have a pervasive effect upon both sleep quantity and quality. Depressed patients tend to have difficulty falling asleep, an increased number of awakenings during the night, early morning awakening, non-restorative sleep, decreased total sleep and disturbing dreams. It is likely that the occurrence of nightmares in depression is associated with changes in REM sleep. Not only is REM latency reduced, but increased duration of REM and rate of rapid eye movements have been reported (see Benca 1994). Some sufferers of depression also report that they are sleepy during the day, and some compensate by taking naps.

It has been suggested that some depression is caused by deficient activity in a range of neurotransmitters. A raised level of monoamine oxidase occurs, which catabolises the neurotransmitters noradrenaline and 5-hydroxytryptamine (5-HT), each of which is involved in sleep onset and maintenance (Colling 1983). This can be corrected by the use of antidepressant drugs, including tricyclics, monoamine oxidase inhibitors and newer drugs. These all increase the rate of monoaminergic nerve transmission in the brain.

SPECIFIC SLEEP DISORDERS

Parasomnias

Within the International Classification of Sleep Disorders (see Ch. 1) parasomnias refer to 'undesirable physical phenomena which occur predominantly during sleep'. These are far less likely to be an issue for nurses than the general complaints of insomnia due to environmental or other influences. However, to be aware of their existence and relative seriousness is a useful addition to knowledge. Several of the most common of these disorders are mentioned below.

Sleepwalking

This disorder is present in between 1–15% of the general population and is more common in children than adults, and in boys than girls. Sleepwalking (somnambulism) begins during SWS. During episodes, the sleepers typically begin by sitting up with their eyes open, pluck at their bedding and then get up and walk around. They may be confused and empty their bladder or bowels. Sleepwalkers are usually uncommunicative, unaware of their surroundings and usually either return to bed spontaneously or lie down and sleep somewhere else. They are often amnesic, either remembering nothing or having only partial memory about the episode. These memories may be of frightening dreams such as being trapped or buried.

The main concern is for the safety of the sleepwalkers and their cohabitees. Some have mistaken windows for doors and injured themselves after walking through them. Others have attacked family members. If somnambulism is frequent, the bed should be moved to the ground floor, and sleepers should ensure that they do not have easy night-time access to knives or other potential weapons.

Sleepwalking usually begins in children under 10 years, and stops by the age of 15. However, it does occur in a few adults. The causes are obscure. In adults it may be indicative of stress or more serious problems. Crisp et al (1990) found that sleepwalkers scored very highly on measures of externally directed hostility, suggesting the possibility of associated psychopathological disorders. Treatment is difficult. Drug therapy, for example with benzodiazepines, has had limited success (e.g. Pedley & Guilleminault 1977, Reid & Gutnik 1980). Behavioural treatment and hypnosis have produced improvement in some individuals (Reid et al 1981).

Sleep terrors (night terrors)

Sleep terrors (or night terrors) are closely related to sleepwalking and also occur during SWS. They are sometimes referred to as incubus attacks in adults, and involve sleep paralysis and hypnagogic hallucinations. They are more common among children, who may emit a terrified scream about an hour after the onset of sleep. This is accompanied by an extremely rapid pulse, sweating and respiratory distress. It is difficult to wake children during night terrors, and usually they calm down by themselves after a few minutes, returning to normal sleep. The vast majority have no memory of it the following morning. The causes of sleep terrors are not known, but adult sufferers have been shown to score highly on anxiety scales (Crisp et al 1990). They occur in emotionally disturbed adults such as those suffering from post-traumatic stress disorder. They may also be a result of head injury or a toxic reaction, including drug side-effects.

Bruxism (teeth grinding)

There are two kinds of sleep-related bruxism; one (diurnal) involves grinding the teeth during both the day and the night, while the other (nocturnal) occurs only during sleep. Diurnal bruxism is thought to be related to stress, and may be treated using biofeedback techniques. The prevalence of nocturnal bruxism is thought to be around 5–20% of the general population. Typically it involves violent, repetitive and episodic grinding of the teeth during sleep. This occurs approximately once per second for a minimum of 4–5 seconds, and often lasts for much longer. Bruxism occurs in all stages of sleep throughout the night.

The cause of nocturnal bruxism is not known, and therefore treatments aim to protect the teeth, for example with a toothguard, rather than to cure the tooth grinding itself. It gradually wears the teeth down, and occasionally the grinder wakes up with a sore jaw. It often creates more of a sleep problem for the bed partner, since it can produce a very loud noise. It tends to increase during stressful periods and gradually diminishes after the age of 40.

Nocturnal enuresis

Nocturnal enuresis in children under 5 is not considered pathological. However, there is no exact age when all children should be dry, since there are normal individual variations in neurological and other development. Wetting usually occurs during SWS. This condition can cause great anxiety and social embarrassment and requires careful assessment and treatment. Most children simply grow out of it. The most common causes of nocturnal enuresis in older children are small bladder capacity, lazy bladder syndrome, wide bladder neck anomaly, urinary tract infection and obstruction. Once the cause has been elicited, appropriate treatment may be commenced. In prolonged cases where the cause is unknown, tricyclic antidepressants have been used to treat the condition, with some success, although it is not understood exactly why.

Organic/intrinsic sleep disorders

Described as organic in ICD-10, or intrinsic in ICSD (see Ch. 1), three conditions, in particular, merit attention because of their prevalence, severity, or contribution to overall levels of insomnia: sleep apnoea; periodic movements in sleep (PMS); and narcolepsy.

Sleep apnoea

Sleep apnoea (spelled with the diphthong in the UK and without, as apnea, in the USA) refers to the temporary cessation of breathing during sleep. Clinically, sleep apnoeas can be divided into three types: obstructive sleep apnoea syndrome (OSAS); central sleep apnoea; and a mixed (obstructive/central) type. Obstructive sleep apnoea syndrome is characterised by a closure of the pharynx during sleep, due partly to a collapse of the supportive pharyngeal muscles, and partly to intrapharyngeal suction during inspiration. This closure is frequently accompanied by loud snoring as the patient attempts to breathe through a progressively narrower pharyngeal lumen. Eventually, negative intrapharyngeal pressure collapses the airway completely, and respiration ceases (in severe cases for up to 1 minute). Respiratory effort continues throughout the apnoeic episode until the patient is aroused (or shifts to a lighter stage of sleep), at which point airflow resumes, often with loud gasps, and the cycle begins again (see Fig. 3.2). For some patients, the number of such arousals per night can be in the hundreds. In severe cases, arterial oxygen saturation (SaO_2) can fall below 85% during apnoeic episodes, only to rise again as breathing resumes. Central sleep apnoea, on the other hand, is due to the respiratory centres in the brainstem producing a reduced drive to breathe; mixed sleep apnoeas appear to combine obstructive and central features.

Obstructive sleep apnoea is certainly the commonest type, and is currently estimated to affect approximately 3.8% of the UK population (Ohayon et al 1997). Since sleep apnoeas tend to take place during stages 1, 2 and REM sleep, the patient is effectively

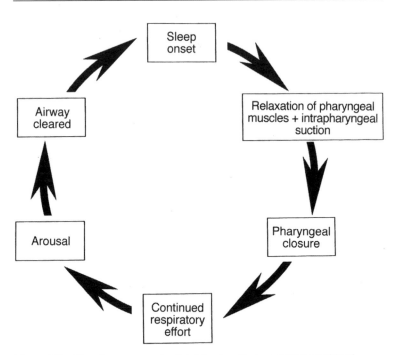

Figure 3.2 The sleep apnoea 'cycle': following sleep onset the combined influence of relaxed pharyngeal muscles and intrapharyngeal suction collapse the airway completely; respiratory effort continues with the patient eventually arousing, or shifting to a lighter stage of sleep; breathing now resumes, blood gasses return to normal, and the patient returns to sleep.

denied access both to deeper sleep stages, and continuous sleep. It is unsurprising, therefore, that the cardinal presenting symptom of OSAS is excessive daytime sleepiness (hypersomnia). This sleepiness may severely impede daytime functioning, including driving and working. In some cases, this somnolence can become highly debilitating, resulting in poor quality of life. Not all OSAS patients, however, are aware of waking during the night, and consequently may not associate their daytime symptoms with the quality of their night-time sleep. Nevertheless, OSAS can also present as insomnia, the direct complaint of degraded sleep quality. Obstructive sleep apnoeas become more common with age, and have been shown to occur in 24% of independently living elderly people (over 65) and 42% of nursing home residents (Ancoli-Israel 1989, Ancoli-Israel et al 1991a). The condition is also associated with obesity, smoking, and alcohol consumption, and can be worsened or precipitated by benzodiazepine hypnotics. Preliminary advice to sufferers, therefore, would include losing weight (if appropriate), giving up smoking, and avoiding alcohol and hypnotics. Invasive treatments, including surgery to remove soft tissues, have shown some success in the management of OSAS (see Powell et al 1994). The most commonly used non-surgical intervention, nasal continuous positive airways pressure (nasal CPAP), maintains the airway by providing, via a special nasal appliance, a physical pressure 'splint' to the pharynx (Popper et al 1986). In clinical practice, all-night CPAP has been reported to dramatically relieve symptoms and improve quality of life in sleep apnoea sufferers (see Stradling & Davis 1997). Nevertheless, Wright et al (1997) suggest the need for further clinical trials to both quantify the advantages of CPAP treatment, and identify the patients who benefit most.

Periodic limb movements (PLM) and restless legs syndrome (RLS)

Restless legs syndrome (RLS) usually occurs late in the evening or while the sufferer is in bed, and is characterised by an unpleasant crawling sensation. This is commonly experienced in the legs, but may also be felt in the muscles of the arms. It is exacerbated by caffeine; and in women it may first appear during pregnancy. In severe cases, RLS may produce emotional disturbances; occasionally it is severe enough to produce depression and suicidal thoughts. The frequency and intensity of this condition varies throughout the patient's lifetime. Its prevalence is not clear but is thought to be over 5% of the general population. The cause is unknown, and it is commonly reported that exercising the affected muscles is the only way of getting rid of it.

Also classified within the ICSD as a cause of both insomnia and excessive daytime sleepiness, PLM is characterised by involuntary limb movements which can occur in all stages of sleep, but tend to predominate in the lighter stages (stages 1 and 2; Montplaisir et al 1994). While movement and positional changes occur throughout normal sleep, four or more consecutive limb movements lasting 0.5–5 seconds (with an inter-movement interval of 4–90 seconds) are regarded as PLM episodes. More than five such episodes per night is considered pathological. PLM increases with age, with an estimated prevalence among elderly people living at home of about 45% (Ancoli-Israel 1991b). Once again, however, not all those showing signs of PLM experience disturbed sleep. Thus, while undoubtedly a cause of disturbed sleep in later life, many of the links between PLM and sleep complaints remain to be explored. Benzodiazepines reduce the arousals, but do not always reduce the leg movements during sleep. Other drugs, such as propoxyphene, baclofen and levodopa may alleviate these conditions.

Narcolepsy

This is a rare but serious sleep disorder, occurring in 4 per 10 000 people. It often develops near puberty, but most symptoms occur between the ages of 15–25. It is thought to result from an imbalance between REM, NREM and wakefulness. Depending on its severity, it may be a mild inconvenience for some, while for others it is extremely debilitating, with excessive sleepiness and daytime sleep attacks being the first symptoms. Later symptoms include cataplexy, abnormal REM sleep patterns, sleep paralysis, and hypnagogic hallucinations, although these are not experienced by all those with narcolepsy all the time.

Cataplexy is perhaps the most widely known symptom, occurring in about 60% of cases. It involves a sudden brief loss of muscle tone usually triggered by emotional responses such as laughter, anger and excitement. The extent is variable, ranging from a slight buckling of the knees to the relaxation of the entire voluntary musculature. The sufferer is aware of what is happening throughout, unlike during a fit. Sleep paralysis is usually associated with great anxiety, disturbing hypnagogic hallucinations and the inability to move any musculature during the process of either falling asleep or waking up. Fortunately, these episodes tend to be brief, lasting for about 10 minutes or so.

The cause of narcolepsy is not known, although there appear to be genetic factors involved (see Guilleminault 1994, p. 549). Behavioural treatments can help with this condition, in particular taking scheduled afternoon naps seems to reduce the incidence of daytime narcoleptic episodes (Garma & Marchand 1994). Other treatments, including the use of stimulant drugs such as ephedrine, or the avoidance of simple sugars in the diet have had some limited success.

CONCLUSIONS

Many different factors, both internal and external to the sleeper, have the potential to interfere with the quality and quantity of sleep. Nurses have an important screening role here, in the identification of patients to whom they can offer advice and support themselves, and those who need to be referred for specialist help. Nurses themselves may be able to give advice on how to reduce the impact of detrimental environmental and behavioural factors on sleep. And they might attempt to create conditions as similar as possible to those of the home environment of a patient who is in hospital. In the following chapters, consideration will be given to how sleep problems may be assessed, and how treatment and support may be delivered.

REFERENCES

Adam K 1980 Dietary habits and sleep after bedtime food, drinks. Sleep 3:47–58
Akiskal H S, Lemmi H, Dickens H et al 1984 Chronic depression. II. Sleep EEG differentiation of primary dysthymic disorders from anxious depression. Journal of Affective Disorders 6: 287–295
Ancoli-Israel S 1989 Epidemiology of sleep disorders. Clinics in Geriatric Medicine 5: 347–362
Ancoli-Israel S et al 1991a Sleep disordered breathing in community dwelling elderly. Sleep 14: 486–495
Ancoli-Israel S, Kripke D F, Klauber M R, Mason W J, Fell R, Kaplan O 1991b Periodic limb movements in sleep in community dwelling elderly. Sleep 14: 496–500
Aparicio R D V, Varela M S M M, Garcia A G, Gonzalez A L, Ruano L, Sanchez A M, Caraco E F 1993 Subjective annoyance caused by environmental noise. Journal of Environmental Pathology, Toxicology and Oncology 12(4): 237–243
Benca R M 1994 Mood disorders. In: Kryger M H, Roth T, Dement W C (eds) Principles and practice of sleep medicine, 2nd edn. W B Saunders, Philadelphia, pp 899–913
Brezinova V, Oswald I 1972 Sleep after bedtime beverage. British Medical Journal 2(5811): 431–433
Brown S L, Salive M E, Pahor M et al 1995 Occult caffeine as a source of sleep problems in an older population. Journal of the American Geriatrics Society 43(8): 860–864
Coleman R M, Roffwarg H P, Kennedy S J 1982 Sleep–wake disorders based on a polysomnographic diagnosis: a national co-operative study. Journal of the American Medical Association 247: 997–1003
Colling J 1983 Sleep disturbances in aging: a theoretic and empiric analysis. Advances in Nursing Science 6: 36–44
Crisp A H, Stonehill E 1973 Aspects of the relationship between sleep and nutrition. A study of 375 psychiatric outpatients. British Journal of Psychiatry 122: 379–394

Crisp A H, Matthews B M, Oakey M, Crutchfield M 1990 Sleepwalking, night terrors and consciousness. British Medical Journal 300: 360–362

Diamond A W 1991 The future development of chronic pain relief. Anaesthesia 46: 83–84

Domzal T, Szczudlik A, Kwasucki J, Zaleska B, Lypka A 1983 Plasma cortisol concentration in patients with different circadian pain rhythm. Pain 17: 67–70

Drewes A M, Nielsen K D, Arendt-Nielsen L, Birket-Smith L, Hansen L M 1997 The effect of cutaneous and deep pain on the encephalogram during sleep – an experimental study. Sleep 20(8): 632–640

Edelstein B A, Keaton-Brasted C, Burg M M 1984 Effects of caffeine withdrawal on nocturnal enuresis, insomnia and behaviour restraints. Journal of Consulting and Clinical Psychology 52: 857–862

Ford D E, Kamerow D B 1989 Epidemiologic study of sleep disturbances and psychiatric disorders. Journal of the American Medical Association 262: 1479–1484

Garma L, Marchand F 1994 Non-pharmacological approaches to the treatment of narcolepsy. Sleep 17(8 suppl): S97–102

Gentili A, Weiner D K, Kuchibhatil M, Edinger J D 1997 Factors that disturb sleep in nursing home residents. Aging Milano 9(3): 207–213

Glyn C L, Lloyd J W, Folkard S 1976 The diurnal variation in perception of pain. Proceedings of the Royal Society of Medicine 69: 369–372

Guilleminault C 1994 Narcolepsy syndrome. In: Kryger M H, Roth T, Dement W C (eds) Principles and practice of sleep medicine, 2nd edn. W B Saunders, Philadelphia, pp 549–561

Hauri P J (Ed) 1992 Sleep disorders. UpJohn Company, Kalamazoo, MI

Haythornthwaite J A, Hegel M T, Kerns R D 1991 Development of a sleep diary for chronic pain patients. Journal of Pain and Symptom Management 6(2): 65–72

Horne J A 1985 Sleep function with particular reference to sleep deprivation. Annals of Clinical Research 17(5): 199–208

Karacan I, Wolff S M, Williams R L, Hursch C J, Webb W B 1968 The effect of fever on sleep and dream patterns. Psychosomatics 9: 331–339

Karacan I, Thornby J I, Anch A M, Booth G H, Williams R L, Salis P J 1976 Dose-related sleep disturbances induced by coffee and caffeine. Clinical Pharmacology and Therapeutics 20: 682–689

Karacan I, Thornby J I, Anch A M, Williams R L 1978 The effects of high ambient temperature on sleep in young men. Sleep Research 7: 171

Kawada T 1995 Effects of traffic noise on sleep: a review. Nippon-Eiseigaku Zasshi 50(5): 932–938

Kendel J, Schmidt-Kessen W 1973 The influence of room temperature on night-time sleep in man (polygraphic night-sleep recordings in the climate chamber). In: Koella W P, Levin P (eds) Sleep. Karger, Basel, pp 423–425

Kostis J B, Rosen R C, Holzer B C et al 1990 CNS side effects of centrally-active antihypertensive agents: a prospective placebo controlled study of sleep, mood state, and cognitive and sexual function in hypertensive males. Psychopharmacology 102: 163–170

Kreuger J M, Majde J A 1995 Cytokines and sleep. International Archives of Allergy and Immunology 106(2): 97–100

Levy A B, Dixon K N, Schmidt H 1987 REM and delta sleep in anorexia nervosa and bulimia. Psychiatry Research 20: 189–197

Levy A B, Dixon K N, Schmidt H 1988 Sleep architecture in anorexia nervosa and bulimia. Biological Psychiatry 23: 99–101

Moja E A, Antonoro E, Cesa-Bianchi M, Gessa G L 1984 Increase in stage 4 sleep after ingestion of a tryptophan-free diet in humans. Pharmacological Research Communications 16(9): 909–914

Montplaisir J, Godbout R, Pelletier G, Warnes H 1994 Restless legs syndrome and periodic movements during sleep. In: Kryger M H, Roth T, Dement W C (eds) Principles and practice of sleep medicine. W B Saunders, Philadelphia, pp 589–597

Morrell S, Taylor R, Lyle D 1997 A review of the health effects of aircraft noise. Australia and New Zealand Journal of Public Health 21(2): 221–236

Muzet A, Libert J-P, Candas V 1984 Ambient temperature and human sleep. Experientia 40: 425–429

Nicholson A N, Stone B M 1987 Influence of back angle on the quality of sleep in seats. Ergonomics 30: 1033–1041

Nivison M E, Endresen I M 1993 An analysis of relationships among environmental noise, annoyance and sensitivity to noise, and the consequences for health and sleep. Journal of Behavioral Medicine 16(3): 257–276

Ohayon M M, Guilleminault C, Priest R, Caulet M 1997 Snoring and breathing pauses during sleep: telephone interview survey of a United Kingdom population sample. British Medical Journal 314: 860–863

Otto E 1973 Physiological analysis of human sleep disturbances induced by noise and increase in room temperature. In: Koella W P, Levin P (eds) Sleep. Karger, Basel, pp 414–418

Pedley J A, Guilleminault W C 1977 Episodic nocturnal wanderings responsive to anticonvulsant drug therapy. Annals of Neurology 2: 30–35

Phillips G D, Cousins M J 1986 Neurological mechanisms of pain and the relationship of pain, anxiety and sleep. In: Cousins M J, Phillips G D (eds) Acute pain management. Churchill Livingstone, New York

Pilowsky I, Crettenden I, Townley M 1985 Sleep disturbances in pain clinic patients. Pain 23: 27–33

Popper R A, Leidlinger M J, Williams A J 1986 Endoscopic observations of the pharyngeal airway during treatment of obstructive sleep apnea with nasal continuous positive airways pressure – a pneumatic splint. Western Journal of Medicine 144: 83–85

Powell N B, Guilleminault C, Wiley R W 1994 Surgical therapy for obstructive sleep apnea. In: Kryger M H, Roth T, Dement W C (eds) Principles and practice of sleep medicine. W B Saunders, Philadelphia, pp 706–721

Prosise G L, Bonnet M H, Berry R B, Dickel M J 1994 Effects of abstinence from smoking on sleep and daytime sleepiness. Chest 105: 1136–1141

Reynolds C F, Shaw P H, Newton T F et al 1983 EEG sleep in outpatients with generalized anxiety: a preliminary comparison with depressed outpatients. Psychiatry Research 8: 81–89

Reid W H, Ahmed I, Leue C A 1981 Treatment of sleepwalking: a controlled study. American Journal of Psychotherapy 85: 27–37

Reid W H, Gutnik B D 1980 case report: treatment of intractable sleepwalking. Psychiatric Journal of the University of Ottawa 5: 86–88

Reite M, Ruddy J, Nagel K 1997 Concise guide to: evaluation and management of sleep disorders. American Psychiatric Press, Washington, p 52

Roehrs T, Zorick F, Roth T 1994 Transient and short-term insomnia. In: Kryger M H, Roth T, Dement W C (eds) Principles and practice of sleep medicine. W B Saunders, Philadelphia, pp 486–493

Roffwarg H P 1979 Diagnostic classification of sleep and arousal disorders. Sleep 2: 1–137

Short R V 1993 Melatonin, hormone of darkness. British Medical Journal 307: 952–953

Singh N A, Clements K M, Fiatarone M A 1997 A randomized controlled trial of the effect of exercise on sleep. Sleep 20(2): 95–101

Sitaram N, Dube S, Jones D et al 1984 Acetylcholine and alpha-adrenergic sensitivity in the separation of depression and anxiety. Psychopathology 17: 24–39

Soldatos C R, Kales J D, Scharf M B, Bixler E O, Kales A 1980 Cigarette smoking associated with sleep difficulty. Science 207: 551–552

Stradling J R, Davis R J O 1997 The unacceptable face of evidence-based medicine. Journal of Evaluation in Clinical Practice 3(2): 99–103

Thompson D R, Sutton T W, Jowett N I, Pohl J E F 1991 Circadian variation in the frequency of onset of chest pain in acute myocardial infarction. British Heart Journal 65: 177–178

Trinder J, Montgomery I, Paxton S J 1988 The effect of exercise on sleep: the negative view. Acta Physiologica Scandinavica 133 (574): 14–20

Vouri I, Urponen H, Hasan J, Partinen M 1988 Epidemiology of exercise effects on sleep. Acta Physiologica Scandinavica 133 (574): 3–7

Wolter T D, Hauri P J, Schroeder D R et al 1996 Effects of 24-hour nicotine replacement on sleep and daytime activity during smoking cessation. Preventive Medicine 25: 601–610

Wright J, Johns R, Watt I, Melville A, Sheldon T 1997 Health effects of obstructive sleep apnoea and the effectiveness of continuous positive airways pressure: a systematic review of the research evidence. British Medical Journal 314: 851–860

Youngstedt S D, O'Connor P J, Disham R K 1997 The effects of acute exercise on sleep: a qualitative synthesis. Sleep 20(3): 203–214

Zepelin H, McDonald C S, Zammit G K 1984 Effects of age on auditory awakening thresholds. Journal of Gerontology 39(3): 294–300

Zulley J 1980 Timing of sleep within the circadian temperature cycle. Sleep Research 9: 282

Zulley J, Schultz H 1980 Sleep and body temperature in free-running sleep wake cycles. In: Popovitch L, Asgian B, Badiu G (eds) Sleep. Karger, Basel, pp 341–344

4

Managing insomnia: a structured approach

Learning outcomes

The previous three chapters have aimed to provide the foundations to sleep management through an improved understanding of normal sleep and insomnia. Before addressing aspects of practical management, this chapter considers the *structure* of an evidence-based approach, and some of the issues which need to be addressed before treatment begins. On completing this chapter you should be able to:

- explain the need for clear role identification in sleep management
- distinguish between the need to *assess* and *monitor* sleep problems
- name three separate therapeutic approaches to the management of insomnia.

INTRODUCTION

One of the more overlooked disadvantages of high-level hypnotic drug prescribing over the past 30 years has been the inhibition of a broader, more flexible response to the management of poor sleep in primary and secondary care settings. As a result, many health care professions are unfamiliar with the issues involved in interacting with (as opposed to simply prescribing for) insomnia (see Morgan 1990). These issues involve aspects of multidisciplinary working, goal setting with patients, and outcome measurement (all relatively neglected in a response dominated by prescribing). In the following sections, then, attention will be drawn briefly to each of these important points.

THE MULTIDISCIPLINARY CONTEXT

As suggested in Chapter 2, sleep problems are frequently complex and multifactorial in origin, crossing specialities and disciplines in both nursing and medicine. It follows, then, that the optimal management of such problems should arise in a multidisciplinary context. Inevitably, however, multidisciplinary approaches to health care problems introduce the issue of professional boundaries and individual skills. In a team, everybody cannot do everything. While the existence of boundaries between different health professionals may be established by training, tradition or the law, recognition of these boundaries often results mainly from practical experience. A nurse, for example, will use experience to judge when palliative responses to pain should give way to a request for prescribed analgesia. Similarly, a general practitioner will use experience to decide when the management of a person's depression should be passed to a psychologist or psychiatrist. Unfortunately, the interdisciplinary management of sleep is less well established. Consequently, individual health care professionals may not only be unaware of what they themselves can offer, but they may also be unaware of what help can be shared.

What can you offer and what can you share?

The approach to sleep problems described in the following chapters includes aspects of health education, behavioural management, psychological treatment and pharmacological therapy. It is up to individual readers to decide which areas of management fall within their own professional boundaries. Having said that, it is also important to emphasise that many of these responses (e.g. health education, pharmacological therapy) are intended to run in parallel, not in series. That is, as new components of management are introduced, earlier components are continued.

As a general rule, less specialised responses (which require lower levels of skill) are introduced early in management, while more specialised responses (which need higher levels of skill) are introduced later. This is illustrated in Figure 4.1, which identifies six non-pharmacological components of treatment. Hypnotic drug therapy can be introduced at any point in management but, unlike the other interventions, should be time-limited. Each of these components is briefly described in Table 4.1, and will be discussed in subsequent chapters. Suffice it to say here that, given the broad range of expertise and experience within nursing, individuals should judge for themselves how much they can offer, and how much they could share. As a guide, Table 4.1 indicates the probable support needs of a UK post-registration nurse without specialised training.

RESPONDING TO INSOMNIA

Before attempting to manage a sleep problem, it is a useful investment of time if the style, aims and details of the approach to be used are first discussed with the patient. It is particularly important, both for the credibility of the nurse, and the well-being of patients, that the goals of management are clearly understood. As will be shown in later chapters, the aim of management is not to cure insomnia, but to improve sleep quality. This can be made clear to the patient in quite positive terms by emphasising the likelihood of improvement (rather than emphasising the likelihood of no cure). This aim can be expressed in another way. Quite often it is the sheer unpredictability of sleep which most impacts upon quality of life in those with a chronic sleep problem – not knowing if they are going to lie awake for hours or fall asleep exhausted. Successful management may not restore perfect sleep, but it will help to make sleeping patterns more reliable. And very often that is enough.

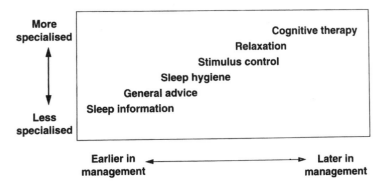

Figure 4.1   Effective responses to insomnia range from less specialised to more specialised interventions (vertical axis), with the more specialised requiring greater nursing skills. It is both rational and economical to offer the less specialised interventions earlier in management, building on these inputs as management develops (horizontal axis).

Table 4.1 An overview of treatment options in the management of insomnia

Response	Description	Support needs of UK post-registration nurse
Hypnotic drugs	CNS depressants which bind to (mostly) benzodiazepine receptors. Modern hypnotics are extremely effective, and are safe in overdose	Not applicable
Sleep information	Information designed to build realistic expectations of sleep (duration, continuity, onset latency, etc.)	Familiarity with information in Chapters 2 and 3. This response could be delivered by a post-registration nurse
General advice	Advice aimed at a broad range of patients, concerning some of the more general aspects of sleep hygiene	Familiarity with information provided in Chapters 3 and 6. This response could be delivered by a post-registration nurse
Sleep hygiene	Advice, based on patient assessment, to encourage behaviours which promote sleep, and discourage behaviours antagonistic to sleep	Information provided in Chapter 6. This response could be delivered by a post-registration nurse
Stimulus control	One of the most effective psychological treatments for insomnia, based on strengthening learned connections between the sleep environment and sleep onset	Information provided in Chapter 7. This response could be delivered by a post-registration nurse. Supervision by an experienced therapist or nurse specialist is recommended
Relaxation techniques	Therapies which promote the relaxed state essential for sleep onset	Information provided in Chapter 8. This response could be delivered by a post-registration nurse. Supervision by an experienced therapist or nurse specialist is recommended
Cognitive therapy	Generic title given to psychological therapies which aim to interrupt links between maladaptive (counterproductive) thoughts and beliefs, and negative behavioural outcomes (e.g. insomnia)	This response could be delivered by a post-registration nurse, but only after additional specialised training. Supervision by a skilled therapist is recommended

It is also important to realise that a problem successfully managed at one point in time can return at another. This, however, serves to illustrate one of the strengths of the structured, flexible approach described here. If put into practice, self-help and psychological strategies equip the patient to deal more effectively with both present and future problems.

Overcoming resistance

The successful management of insomnia is usually impossible without the cooperation and effort of the patient. Nevertheless, active participation in treatment, particularly when it means doing things which are temporarily inconvenient, can meet with resistance. Keep in mind that, for many years, sleeping tablets have dominated the management of insomnia and that active participation in management may, to some patients, seem rather unorthodox. Naturally, the patient has the right to choose not to cooperate; behavioural approaches do not suit everybody. If, however, you wish to offer encouragement, then it might be useful to point out: (a) that if cooperating is really no worse than the problem, then the client has nothing to lose; and (b) that for a number of reasons sleep problems may get worse over time, and that a little inconvenience now may prevent a lot of inconvenience later. It is relevant to note here that, when offered a choice between pharmacological and psychological interventions, patients consistently rate psychological approaches as more acceptable (Morin et al 1992).

Insomnia: a structured response

The overall therapeutic strategy described in subsequent chapters is based on the sequence: assessment; intervention; outcome measurement. It is a sequence well established in the psychological management of insomnia (e.g. Espie 1991, Lacks 1987, Morin 1993), and increasingly recommended for multidisciplinary management (Lader 1992, National Medical Advisory Committee 1994). Within this strategy there is another guiding principle: manage the simpler issues first. In this way, the response can build up in a logical and practical way. If sufficient improvement is obtained with relatively simple interventions, the more complex (and the more time-

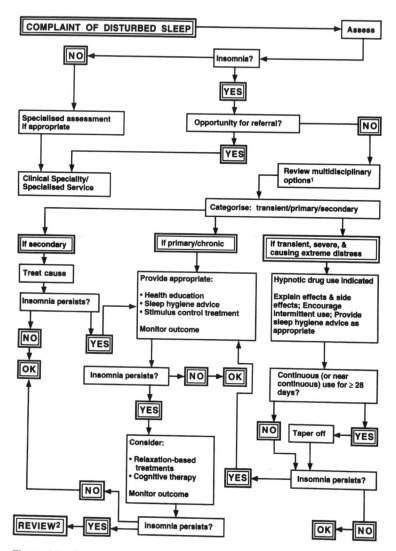

Figure 4.2 Sleep management in a multidisciplinary context. The flow-chart summarises and organises the major decisions and options which need to be considered. To avoid episode repetitions, 'OK' should be interpreted as 'encourage continued sleep hygiene'.

[1]Options and resources may vary widely; this review should aim to optimise available resources.

[2]This review should include attention to the initial diagnosis, reappraisal of possible underlying causes of the present insomnia, appropriateness of the original treatment goals, and the degree of treatment adherence.

consuming and expensive) interventions can be avoided. There is another reason for responding in this way. Sometimes different factors underlying insomnia cause problems only when they act together. The excessive consumption of coffee (which, as a stimulant, acts to promote arousal and antagonise sleep onset) may become a problem only if some further factor (pain, illness, anxiety) starts to disturb sleep. A broad systematic approach to management can help to interrupt such interactions, and optimise improvement. Some of the major decisions and options involved in sleep management are summarised in the flow chart shown in Figure 4.2. It is possible that some of the options described will not be available to all health care professionals. Nevertheless, following the principles of flexibility, multidisciplinarity, and monitored outcomes implicit in this algorithm, the delivery of effective management can be optimised.

Guiding the development of treatment is *outcome measurement*. Continued throughout management, this monitoring is really a form of serial assessment which enables both the patient and the professionals to quantify the impact of intervention. Interestingly, such monitoring can also become therapeutic, as tangible evidence of improvement reinforces the patients' (and the professionals') efforts. The first component of management, assessment, is described in the next chapter.

REFERENCES

Espie C A 1991 The psychological treatment of insomnia. Wiley, Chichester
Lacks P 1987 Behavioral treatment for persistent insomnia. Pergamon, New York
Lader M (ed) 1992 The medical management of insomnia in general practice.
    Royal Society of Medicine Round Table Series 28, Royal Society of Medicine,
    London
Morgan K 1990 Hypnotics in the elderly: what's the problem? Geriatric Medicine
    20(6): 9
Morin C M 1993 Insomnia – psychological assessment and management.
    Guilford Press, New York
Morin C M, Gaulier B, Barry T, Kowatch R A 1992 Patients' acceptance of
    psychological and pharmacological therapies for insomnia. Sleep 15: 302–305
National Medical Advisory Committee 1994 The management of anxiety and
    insomnia. HMSO, Edinburgh

The assessment of sleep

Learning outcomes

This chapter deals with the first practical steps towards evidence-based management – the assessment and monitoring of sleep. The aims and rationale of sleep assessment are first introduced, issues relating to assessment are discussed, and methods for assessing sleep and insomnia are then presented. Since sleep is increasingly forming part of the nursing research agenda, the chapter includes a description of assessment instruments with both clinical and research utility.
On completing this chapter you should be able to:

- name four aspects of sleep which might usefully be assessed in clinical practice
- describe differences between subjective estimates and objective measurements of sleep latency, and total sleep time
- construct a simple sleep diary
- name five aspects of sleep history which could usefully be collected on admission for long-stay patients.

INTRODUCTION

Fundamental to the evidence-based management of sleep and insomnia is the need to conduct valid assessments of sleep itself. Both the aim, and the complexity of such assessments show considerable variations. Some approaches to assessment screen for causes of sleep difficulties. Other approaches are more appropriate for monitoring sleep in order to gauge improvements resulting from nursing or other interventions. All of these assessments may include descriptions of the circumstances preceding sleep, the sleep itself (or the lack of it) and the after-effects of that sleep. In addition to the content and emphasis of the assessment, the role of the assessor may also vary from situation to situation. Assessment may form part of an individual nurse's treatment plan for a given patient, or it may form part of a team effort. Assessments may be used by those monitoring patients undergoing treatments likely to disrupt sleep, or by those monitoring the outcome of a specific sleep intervention. As suggested in Chapter 1, in both primary and secondary care settings, nurses are well placed to take on part of the management of sleep difficulties, and to take the initiative in sleep assessment and monitoring. While the broad aim of this chapter is to introduce methods for assessment, important issues concerning the validity and reliability of sleep information will also be considered.

ASSESSING SLEEP: OBSERVATIONS AND REPORTS

There are many different approaches to the assessment of sleep, each addressing different aspects of sleep–wake functioning, or reflecting differing methodologies. Some of these may be used in everyday clinical situations, while others are more suitable for research, or sophisticated differential diagnosis. Examples of different methodologies, and different target phenomena, are provided in Tables 5.1 and 5.2 respectively. In nursing practice, clinical/subjective approaches to sleep assessment tend to predominate, either as nurse observations, or as some kind of patient self report. Both have been evaluated in research studies.

Accuracy of nurse observations, reports and records

The role of nurses in assessing the sleep of their patients varies according to the setting. Community nurses are unlikely to monitor sleep routinely, and will probably identify only those cases where extreme problems are volunteered. However, ensuring that patients sleep as well as possible is a central function of the hospital nurse. For the most part, hospital nurses have two ways of obtaining information about patients' sleep: by observing patients during the night and forming an opinion about the length and quality of sleep; and by asking patients about their sleep the following morning.

Table 5.1   Assessment of various aspects of sleep–wake functioning

Aspect of sleep–wake functioning	What can be assessed
Characteristics of sleep	Time at which the individual settled down to sleep
	Time taken to fall asleep in minutes (sleep onset latency (SOL))
	Time of morning waking
	Time spent asleep during the night
	Number of times awakened during the night
	Time spent awake during the night (wakefulness after sleep onset (WASO))
	Pattern of sleep stages throughout the night
	Body movements during sleep
	Arousal thresholds
	Time spent napping during the day
Impact of sleep	Satisfaction with sleep quality/quantity
	Feeling of being refreshed on waking
	Ability to concentrate during the day
	Sleepiness during the day
	Mood states

Table 5.2   Methods for assessing sleep–wake functioning

Approach	Aspect of sleep	
	Sleep	After-effects of sleep
Clinical/subjective	Sleep diaries	Sleep diaries
	Subjective rating scales	Subjective rating scales
	Visual analogue scales	Visual analogue scales
	Interviews	Interviews
	Observation	–
Academic/objective	Polysomnography (electroencephalogram (EEG), electromyogram (EMG) and electrooculogram (EOG))	–
	Actigraphy (body movements)	–
	Arousal thresholds	–
	–	Vigilance
	–	Multiple sleep latency test (sleepiness)

There are problems associated with each of these approaches. Observation is difficult to do accurately, and patients' reports of sleep are often polite 'very well, thank you' responses which may or may not bear any resemblance to their experiences. Consequently, nurses' written records of sleep tend to lack validity and accuracy.

Observation

Observational methods of quantifying sleep have been widely used in research studies. At best, observation may identify two qualitatively different states of consciousness: wakefulness and sleep. Intermittent observations of the sleeper, for example every hour during the night, are of limited use since the sleeper may wake up between observations without this being noticed. Furthermore, it is not possible to distinguish either between dozing and deep restorative sleep, or between the time of initially falling asleep and of finally waking up with any precision. Some of the problems can be overcome by using continuous observation, perhaps by using a video camera or closed-circuit television (Johns et al 1969). The main point, however, is that it is not always possible to assess level of consciousness accurately, simply by looking at the sleeper. It is relevant to note that many hospital patients pretend to be asleep when nurses approach them during the night, since they perceive the nurses as being busy and do not wish to 'be a nuisance' (Closs 1992, Dodds 1980).

Research which has compared nurses' observation-based estimates of sleep duration with sleep as assessed using polysomnography have, for the most part, been undertaken in intensive care settings. Aurell & Elmqvist (1985) found that nurses made inaccurate estimates of patients' sleep duration, often overestimating by several hours. Other similar studies showed rather better results, where reasonable agreement was found between nurses' assessments and the corresponding polysomnogram (Edwards & Schuring 1993, Fontaine 1989). However, it might be expected that the high staff/patient ratio in an ICU would allow nurses more frequent opportunities to observe (every 5–15 minutes preferably), greater familiarity with their patients and better lighting conditions making it easier actually to see patients. In general hospital wards, this may be far more difficult. In non-ICU hospital settings, nurse ratings have been found consistently to overestimate the sleep of hospital patients (Kupfer et al 1970, Weiss et al 1973). Indeed, in a comparison of 26 studies in which the sleep of elderly people had been either observed or polysomnographically recorded, direct observations were found to yield the highest estimates of total sleep time (Regestein et al 1987).

Nursing records

Over 20 years ago, a study of the Kardexes of more than 700 medical and surgical inpatients showed that pain and sleep were the least well recorded categories of care (Georgopolous & Jackson 1970). This lack of documentation has been confirmed more recently. Out of 200 surgical patients who were interviewed about their previous night's sleep, less than half had any mention of sleep quality and less than 10% had any mention of the duration of their sleep in their nursing notes (Closs 1992). Other studies have also shown that sleep is sparsely and infrequently documented (Edéll-Gustafsson et al 1994, Ehnfors & Smedby 1993). Sleep assessment seems rarely to be undertaken systematically, more often being based on random observations and equally random recordings. Suggestions for the systematic assessment and documentation of hospital patients' sleep are given towards the end of this chapter.

It is difficult to know why such a fundamental aspect of human functioning is apparently such a low priority for nurses. The assessment of intangible experiences, such as pain and sleep is not easy and nurses need to give patients an opportunity to give an account of their sleep. This should be done in such a way that patients feel that the enquiry is genuine and the nurse attaches importance to what they say. Consequently, a ritualistic question such as 'did you sleep well last night?' almost obliges a response such as 'yes thank you', regardless of patients' actual experiences. More open questions which provide an opening for patients to give detail about their sleep such as 'how did you sleep last night? did you have any problems?' are more useful.

It may also be that documentation is sparse because nurses exchange information about patients' sleep verbally, or maybe there is an assumption that patients are asleep unless it is blatantly obvious that they are not. It may also be due to a lack of knowledge about what should usefully be documented as well as a lack of a standardised language with which to describe the various aspects of sleep and its disturbance. Equipping nurses with the necessary concepts and language might improve matters.

How accurate are sleepers' reports?

Sleep is a very private experience and subjective reports provide descriptions of sleep as it is experienced by the sleeper. Broadly, these reports may be of two kinds: experiences of sleep quality; and estimates of sleep quantity. As regards sleep quality, it should be emphasised that the experience of sleep is accessible only to the individual sleepers. Only they know whether their sleep has been restful and refreshing. In addition, criteria for a 'good night's sleep' are also, to some extent, personal. Whether individuals sleep for 2 hours per night, or for 10 hours per night, if they awake, satisfied with their sleep quality, and can function efficiently during the day, then their sleep may be considered satisfactory (or normal for them).

But how accurate are sleepers' estimates of sleep quantity? Simple questions asking subjects with and without insomnia for assessments of their own sleep duration, or the number of awakenings during the night have not always produced accurate information (Carskadon et al 1976, Frankel et al 1976, Monroe 1967). Comparing subjective and EEG data from groups of poor sleepers, Carskadon et al (1976) found that most consistently underestimated the length of time spent asleep and overestimated the time taken to get to sleep. Interestingly, a degree of internal consistency exists in such estimates, since individuals, both with and without insomnia, tend systematically to underestimate their total sleep. As Frankel et al (1976) commented: 'Even though insomniacs consistently overestimated their sleeplessness, their polysomnographic sleep patterns could be predicted from their subjective estimates'. Similar conclusions were reached in the comparisons of self-reported good and poor sleepers conducted by Monroe (1967) and Adam et al (1986). Both studies found that poor sleepers did indeed sleep (up to half an hour) less that good sleepers, with Adam et al (1986) also observing that poor sleepers nevertheless overestimated their sleeplessness. To some extent, these discrepancies may reflect fundamentally different experiences of sleep among good and poor sleepers. In an EEG study, for example, Borkovec et al (1981) found that when good and poor sleepers were woken in the fifth consecutive minute of stage 2 sleep, poor sleepers were more likely to report that they had been awake. It seems, then, that individuals can provide estimates of their sleep patterns which correlate with (but that differ from) objective measurements, and are very sensitive to changes in their own normal sleep.

ASSESSING AND MONITORING PROBLEM SLEEP

The methods of assessing sleep presented so far have been concerned almost entirely with describing (rather than measuring) sleep and its after-effects. Where patients actively seek help for sleep problems (or, in the judgement of a health care professional, might benefit from help for a sleep problem), then a more formal approach to assessment is needed. In such cases, more information about the precise nature of sleep difficulties is required, so that the nurse can either refer patients on to others, or deal with the problem him/herself.

Aims of assessment

Where a sleep problem has presented, and where treatment is anticipated, formal assessment procedures meet three distinct aims. First, assessment will provide important background information (history) and help to clarify the current problem; second, assessment should aim to identify specific targets for intervention; and third, early assessment provides an essential baseline against which subsequent outcomes are measured.

General assessments

A simple questionnaire which produces a general picture of sleep and the sleepers' perceptions of the causes of any problems can be used as a first step. An example of such a questionnaire which might be used either by hospital or community nurses in order to produce a picture of an individual's usual sleep is shown in Figure 5.1. Such questionnaires are useful for providing an overall description of an individual's usual daily pattern of sleep. More detailed information may be needed in some cases, and a sleep history questionnaire designed to identify causal factors is shown in Figure 5.2.

Below are some questions concerning your sleep. Please answer all the questions. If your times for going to bed and so on vary greatly, give ranges (e.g. 10–11 p.m., 30–60 min).

1	For how long do you usually sleep at night?	
2	After settling down, how long does it usually take you to fall asleep?	
3	How often do you wake up too early in the morning? (tick one)	Never ☐ Seldom ☐ Sometimes ☐ Often ☐ All the time ☐
4	Do you usually wake up during the night?	Yes ☐ No ☐
5	If 'Yes': what usually awakes you? (answer in your own words)	
6	How many times (on average) do you awake each night?	
7	For how long are you awake on each of these occasions?	
8	At what time do you usually go to bed?	
9	At what time do you usually wake up (in the morning)?	
10	At what time do you usually get up?	
11	How refreshed do you usually feel when you wake up in the morning (tick one)?	Very refreshed ☐ Quite refreshed ☐ Unrefreshed ☐ Tired ☐ Shattered ☐
12	In general, how much sleep do you think a person your age needs?	
13	How long have you had your present sleep problem?	

Figure 5.1 A simple sleep questionnaire (source: Morgan & Gledhill 1991).
(cont'd on page 77)

14	What do you think is the cause of your present sleep problem? (answer in your own words)	
15	Have you ever had serious trouble with your sleep in the past?	Yes ☐ No ☐
16	Have you gained or lost weight in the last few months? (tick one)	Yes I have gained weight ☐ Yes I have lost weight ☐ No, I am about the same ☐
17	Before the present problem how would you have described yourself? (tick one)	A very good sleeper ☐ A good sleeper ☐ An average sleeper ☐ A poor sleeper ☐ A very poor sleeper ☐
18	How would you describe yourself now?	A very good sleeper ☐ A good sleeper ☐ An average sleeper ☐ A poor sleeper ☐ A very poor sleeper ☐
19	Do you usually take a nap during the day?	Yes ☐ No ☐
20	When do you usually nap? (give length of each nap)	
	Thank you for completing this questionnaire	

Figure 5.1 *(cont'd)*

Name ——————————————— Date ———————————

1. How many nights per week do you usually have difficulty falling asleep? ____

2. On nights when you *do have* difficulty falling asleep, how many *minutes* does it usually take you to fall asleep after going to bed? ——————

3. On nights when you *do not have* difficulty getting to sleep, how many *minutes* does it usually take you to fall asleep after going to bed? ————

4. Do you ever wake up in the middle of the night and have difficulty falling back to sleep?   YES   NO

   a. If yes, about how many nights does this happen each week? ——————————————

   b. On average, how many times do you wake up each night? ————————

   c. How many minutes does it usually take you to get back to sleep each time you awaken? ————————————————————

5. How often do you wake up early in the morning, before your scheduled wake time, and are unable to return to sleep? ——————————————

6. On nights when you have insomnia, approximately how long do you sleep each night? ——————————————

7. How long have you had a sleep problem? ————————————————

8. How long would you like to be able to sleep each night? ——————————

9. Is your sleep problem sometimes worse than other times?   YES   NO
   If yes, explain ————————————————————————
   ——————————————————————————————————————

10. Why do you think you have a sleep problem? ——————————————
    ——————————————————————————————————————

11. Was the onset of your problem related to any specific event?   YES   NO
    If yes, describe ———————————————————————
    ——————————————————————————————————————

12. Do you sleep better when you are away from home?   YES   NO

13. What do you do when you can't sleep? ———————————————
    ——————————————————————————————————————

14. When you try to sleep, is it hard for you to turn off your mind?   YES   NO

15. Have you been under stress more than usual recently?   YES   NO
    If yes, explain ————————————————————————
    ——————————————————————————————————————

16. Are you the kind of person who tends to worry a lot?   YES   NO

Figure 5.2   Sleep history questionnaire (source: Lacks 1987).
(cont'd on page 79)

17. How often is your sleep disturbed by environmental factors such as traffic, neighbours, or family members? _____

18. Is your bedroom adequately dark at night?   YES   NO

19. On weekends or your days off, do you sleep more than an hour later than your usual wake up time?   YES   NO

20. How many times per week do you take naps? _____

21. Are you on a weight loss program?   YES   NO

22. Do you engage in some kind of physical exercise?   YES   NO

    If yes, describe the time, frequency and time of day _____

23. How many cups or glasses of caffeinated beverages (e.g. coffee, tea or cola) do you drink in a day?

              coffee   tea   cola

24. How many days a week do you drink caffeinated beverages after 4 p.m.? ___

25. Do you take any medications that contain caffeine or stimulants (e.g. allergy medication or painkillers)   YES   NO

    a. If yes, what medication and dose? _____

    b. How often do you usually take it? _____

    c. How soon before bed do you take it? _____

26. How often do you use alcohol to aid sleep? _____

27. How many cigarettes a day do you smoke? _____

28. Does difficulty sleeping ever affect your mood during the day?   YES   NO

29. Would you describe yourself as an especially nervous person?   YES   NO

30. Estimate how many nightmares you have had in the past year _____

31. How often and what amounts of alcohol do you drink? _____

32. Have you ever been treated or hospitalised for mental, emotional, drug or alcohol problems?   YES   NO

33. Does difficulty sleeping affect your functioning during the day?   YES   NO

    If yes, describe how it affects your functioning _____

34. Do you snore?   YES   NO

35. Do you ever wake up in the night and feel unable to breathe?   YES   NO

36. Do your legs ever jerk repeatedly or feel restless after you go to bed at night?   YES   NO

37. Do you ever work the night shift? (11 p.m.–7 a.m.)   YES   NO

38. Do you work a rotating or split shift?   YES   NO

    If yes, please describe _____

Figure 5.2   *(cont'd on page 80)*

39. Have you recently taken any prescription or over-the-counter medication for sleeping problems?   YES   NO

    a. If yes, what medication and amount are you taking? _____

    b. How many nights a week do you usually take this medication? _____

    c. How long have you been taking sleeping medication? _____

40. Are you currently taking any other medication?   YES   NO

    a. If yes, what medication is it? _____

    b. What illness was it prescribed for? _____

41. Do you have any other physical problems or illnesses?   YES   NO

    If yes, describe _____

42. Have you ever been hospitalised during the past 10 years?   YES   NO

    If yes, please describe _____

43. Have you ever had any convulsions or significant head injury?   YES   NO

    If yes, please describe _____

44. How many times per night do you wake up to use the bathroom? _____

45. How many nights per week do you have indigestion or heartburn? _____

46. Have you previously received treatment for sleeping problems?   YES   NO

    If yes, describe _____

47. Have you tried any self-help remedies for your sleeping problems?   YES   NO

    If yes, describe _____

48. Would you be willing to devote 30 minutes per day to a program of treatment to improve your sleep?   YES   NO

Figure 5.2   *(cont'd)*

The Sleep History Questionnaire (Lacks 1987) comprises 48 questions which focus on health and lifestyle. These cover the following seven categories of information about sleep:

- description of the symptoms, extent and duration of insomnia (Q1–7)
- psychological contributing factors (Q8–16)
- sleep hygiene (Q17–27)
- psychopathology (Q28–32)
- organic sleep pathology (Q33–39)
- serious medical problems (Q40–45)
- previous treatment for insomnia (Q46–48).

Questions 8–27 delineate those areas of sleep difficulty which fall within the province of the nurse, namely psychological factors, environmental factors and sleep hygiene. Interventions designed to deal with these problems are described in subsequent chapters. Problems falling outside these categories, i.e. those with psychopathology, organic pathology or serious medical problems, would need more specialised help.

Monitoring sleep

Two characteristics of insomnia are strongly emphasised in all of the diagnostic systems described in Chapter 1: the impact of insomnia on daytime functioning; and the extension of insomnia over weeks and months. Since both characteristics can vary over time, both require serial (i.e. repeated) assessments. Serial assessment usually takes the form of self-completed daily ratings. Such ratings, commenced at the initial interview, and continued throughout treatment and follow-up periods, meet all three aims of assessment (above), providing valuable outcome information used to monitor and adjust management. A variety of serial assessment methods are available, including visual analogue scales, subjective rating scales, questionnaires, interviews and sleep diaries.

Visual analogue scales

One of the simplest subjective methods is the visual analogue scale. A 100 mm horizontal line with opposing statements at each end, e.g. 'best sleep ever' at one end and 'worst night ever' at the other (Fig. 5.3) is presented to the patient who is asked to place a mark on the line in a position corresponding to his or her perception of the previous night's sleep (with a mark in the centre denoting an average night).

The distance of that mark along the line may then be measured in mm, providing a numerical value for satisfaction for each night. Each subject creates his or her own internalised scale which is extremely sensitive to change and therefore particularly useful for serial assessments (Oswald 1980). A research question such as

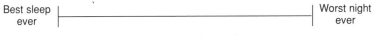

Figure 5.3   Visual analogue scale for monitoring sleep.

'How does the sleep satisfaction of routine surgical patients vary over the duration of admission to hospital' could usefully be addressed using this approach. A possible disadvantage of this particular method is that it is conceptually difficult for some people. In particular, older people sometimes find it difficult to understand. Nevertheless, visual analogue scales have been successfully employed in a number of studies (Bond & Lader 1974, Hindmarch et al 1977, Zealley & Aitken 1969) and have proved particularly useful in the assessment of hypnotic drugs.

Subjective rating scales

Many different types of measure of mood state have been devised, assessing depression, vigour and lethargy. It appears, however, that sleepiness is the only aspect of mood which is consistently and systematically affected by changes in sleep. One of the most sensitive of these types of scales is the Stanford Sleepiness Scale (SSS) designed by Hoddes et al (1972) to quantify levels of subjective sleepiness levels. The SSS utilises a seven-point scale of equal intervals ranging from 1 (very alert) to 7 (excessively sleepy). Several descriptions are used, including 1 (feeling active and vital; alert; wide awake) to 7 (almost in reverie; sleep onset soon; lost in struggle to remain awake). The SSS is sensitive to partial as well as total sleep deprivation, and ratings correlate well with polysomnograph recordings. While the SSS assesses feelings of sleepiness at a particular time, another test has been devised to measure the general level of daytime sleepiness. This is the Epworth Sleepiness Scale (Johns 1991). This scale is brief and easy to complete, and is increasing in popularity.

Subjective rating scales are inexpensive and simple to use, producing relevant and useful information when assessing sleep satisfaction in, for example, cardiac patients. It might be possible to implement more effective schedules for physical and psychological rehabilitation by studying variations in subjective sleepiness throughout the day. Little effort is required by the patient to use such a scale.

Questionnaires

Self-administered questionnaires may be used in order for subjects to answer specific questions about their sleep patterns. These are usually highly structured. For example, a question such as 'what time did you wake up this morning?' is followed by a range of possible answers such as:

1. Before 5 a.m.   ☐
2. 5 a.m.–5.59 a.m.   ☐
3. 6 a.m.–6.59 a.m.   ☐
4. 7 a.m.–7.59 a.m.   ☐
5. 8 a.m.–8.59 a.m.   ☐
6. 9 a.m. or later   ☐

The respondent is simply required to tick the appropriate box. The sensitivity of such instruments may be adjusted by changing the intervals from hourly (as above) to half-hourly, or whatever time intervals are appropriate to the clinical or research question.

More detailed questionnaires have been devised which ask for precise answers to questions such as 'What time did you settle down in bed ready to go to sleep last night?' and 'What time did you wake up this morning?'. Webb (1965) found that this method was reliable on test–retest administrations of the questionnaire, that is when the questions were answered on several different occasions, the subjects gave the same response each time. Occasionally, some practical problems may be encountered, such as the presence of an intravenous infusion sited in the dominant hand or arm, or wrist fractures which could make it difficult to write. Reading might also present difficulties, where bulky facial dressings or inconveniently positioned nasogastric tubes may make it awkward for patients to wear their spectacles. It is important to be sensitive to the possibility that some patients may never have learned to read or write, and may refuse to complete such a questionnaire in order to cover up this fact. Finally, those who are tired, in pain or depressed may be reluctant to respond to the extra demand of completing a questionnaire.

Repeated interviews

These can be structured in much the same way as questionnaires, but may be more appropriate for use with hospital patients who might have difficulty in reading or writing, either due to their illness or otherwise, as mentioned above. This method enables the interviewer to clarify questions if necessary and to ensure that no data are missing, these being major advantages when compared with the use of self-administered questionnaires. One disadvantage is that it is more time-consuming. An example of such an interview was provided by Dodds (1980).

Daily sleep diaries

Daily diaries to monitor sleep quality and quantity are now extensively used in the assessment and management of insomnia, and have become standard in psychological research and practice (Espie 1991, Lacks 1987, Morin 1993). When compared with 24-hour ambulatory polysomnography, sleep diaries have shown high levels of reliability and acceptability (Rogers et al 1993). Among hypnotic drug users in primary care settings, adherence has been found to be high in controlled studies (Espie et al 1988, McClusky et al 1991, Morin 1993, Tomeny & Morgan 1990). In the UK, the practicality and utility of these measures has led to expert recommendations for their use in primary care clinical practice in the management of insomnia (see Lader 1992, National Medical Advisory Committee 1994).

There are many different formats of sleep diary possible and the most appropriate should be selected on the basis of the particular sleep problem being investigated. Three examples are shown here: one providing an overview of sleep quality and quantity (Fig. 5.4); one which focuses on quantities of sleep and wakefulness (Fig. 5.5); and finally, one which is concerned more with the quality of sleep and its after-effects (Fig. 5.6). Completed over a period of weeks, the diary shown in Figure 5.4 can provide a clear sequential representation of basic aspects of sleep (see Fig. 7.2, p. 115). If more emphasis on sleep and wakefulness is required, the format suggested by Rogers et al (1993) may be more useful (Fig. 5.5). An example of a diary which has more emphasis on the quality of sleep and its after-effects has been suggested by Lacks (1987; Fig. 5.6). Although some of the information required is similar, more details in subjective reports such as physical tension and mental activity are required.

Diaries may be returned by post to the agency conducting the assessment either singly (this encourages independent daily ratings), or in batches. Of course, patients need to be motivated to complete diary entries on a daily basis, otherwise recordings are liable to be missed. For this reason, the information being collected should be as brief as possible. Sleep diaries can be used over long periods and are therefore especially useful for monitoring community-based patients with sleep difficulties. However, sleep diaries may not be appropriate for acutely ill patients who have relatively short stays in hospital, since their sleep disturbance is usually a direct result of their acute episode, and once they recover, their sleep returns to normal.

Name		Date
1	At what time did you go to bed last night?	
2	At what time did you settle down to sleep?	
3	How long did it take you to fall asleep?	
4	How many times did you wake up?	
5	What woke you up?	
6	For how long do you think you were awake on each of these occasions?	
7	At what time did you finally wake up?	
8	How did you feel when you woke up this morning? (tick one)	Refreshed and alert ☐ Alert but not at peak ☐ Tired ☐ Absolutely shattered ☐
9	At what time did you get up?	
10	How would you rate last night's sleep? (tick one)	Very good ☐ Good ☐ Average ☐ Poor ☐ Very poor ☐
11	What medicines did you take yesterday?	
12	How much alcohol did you drink yesterday?	

Figure 5.4 A simple sleep diary (source: Morgan & Gledhill 1991).

Subject No. _____

Diary
1. Carry this diary with you at all times during the next 24 hours and write down all your activities.
2. You should record something in each block. The hours are written in the left-hand column and each block represents a quarter of an hour. If you took longer than 15 minutes to do something, just indicate that by drawing an arrow (→) into the next block. Do not worry about recording activities that take only a few minutes; just write down those that took up more than half the time in each 15-minute period.
3. Indicate any sleep periods by shading in the blocks.

	0–15 Minutes	16–30 Minutes	31–45 Minutes	46–60 Minutes
6–7 p.m.				
7–8 p.m.				
8–9 p.m.				
9–10 p.m.				
10–11 p.m.				
11–12 a.m.				
12–1 a.m.				
1–2 a.m.				
2–3 a.m.				
3–4 a.m.				
4–5 a.m.				
5–6 a.m.				
6–7 a.m.				
7–8 a.m.				
8–9 a.m.				
9–10 a.m.				
10–11 a.m.				
11–12 p.m.				
12–1 p.m.				
1–2 p.m.				
2–3 p.m.				
3–4 p.m.				
4–5 p.m.				
5–6 p.m.				

Figure 5.5 Daily sleep record (source: Rogers 1993).

Name _____ Date _____

1. How many minutes did it take you to fall asleep last night? _____

2. How many times did you awaken during the night? _____

3. Please record how long you were awake (in minutes) for each occurrence listed above in question 2.

_____   _____   _____

_____   _____   _____

_____   _____   _____

4. What is the total number of hours and minutes you slept last night? _____

5. How difficult was it for you to fall asleep last night?

1	2	3	4	5
Not very difficult				Extremely difficult

6. How rested do you feel this morning?

1	2	3	4	5
Very rested				Poorly rested

7. Rate the quality of last night's sleep.

1	2	3	4	5
Excellent				Very poor

8. What was your level of physical tension when you went to bed last night?

1	2	3	4	5
Extremely relaxed				Extremely tense

9. Rate your level of mental activity when you went to bed last night.

1	2	3	4	5
Very quiet				Very active

10. How well do you think you were functioning yesterday?

1	2	3	4	5
Very well				Very poorly

Please fold, secure and mail daily

Figure 5.6 A daily sleep diary combining questions and scales (source: Lacks 1987).

The assessment of sleep in hospital

Special issues relating to difficulties involved in sleeping in hospital are discussed in some detail in Chapter 12. Both the screening and monitoring of sleep may be undertaken in hospital settings. A sleep history may be taken on admission, and subsequently morning assessments of the previous night's sleep may be made. In the majority of situations, asking the patient to describe his or her sleep is the best approach.

Sleep history on admission

A description of an individual's usual sleep pattern at home provides a baseline from which to assess the effect of being in hospital. It can also provide information on individual requirements concerning bedtime rituals and preferred environmental conditions. Figure 5.7 shows the kind of questions which would produce this information. For many people, being able to go through their usual routines in the late evening and just before going to bed is of considerable importance. How they prepare themselves for sleep, and their preferred environment for sleep are also worth recording if it is possible that these items could be accommodated. Questions covering these topics are shown in Figure 5.8.

Not only could a sleep history include information about bedtime rituals, time of going to bed and rising, number of awakenings, preferred environmental conditions, drugs and alcohol use, but also tobacco and caffeine use, psychological, medical and neurological conditions, and family history of sleep disorders. It would only be useful to elicit all of this information for those likely to have long stays in hospital. For those who are likely to have a short stay, the most pertinent information would be concerned with how to provide them with the best possible conditions for sleeping.

Daily assessment

The memory of sleep fades rapidly, so it is important to ask patients about their previous night's sleep first thing in the morning. Many patients do not like to complain, feeling that they are a nuisance, or that they do not want to bother busy nurses. Sleep assessments should be designed to ensure that patients are

Usual sleep pattern at home
1. What time do you usually settle down for the night?
2. About what time do you usually fall asleep at night?
3. About how many minutes does it usually take you to fall asleep?
4. How many hours sleep do you usually have at night?
5. How many times do you usually wake up during the night?
6. What wakes you during the night (if anything)?
7. What time do you usually wake up in the morning?
8. How well do you usually sleep throughout the night at home?   Very well ☐   Fairly well ☐   Not very well ☐   Not at all ☐
9. Do you usually nap during the day at home?   Yes ☐   No ☐   If yes, when?   For how long?
10. Do you usually take any medicines to help you sleep at home?   Yes ☐   No ☐   If yes, specify:

Figure 5.7   Questions for a simple sleep history on admission.

able to give an honest report of their night's sleep. Several question-naires have been designed and validated for the assessment of sleep in hospital. These include the St Mary's Hospital Sleep Questionnaire (Ellis et al 1981) and the Snyder-Halpern Verran Sleep Inventory (Snyder-Halpern & Verran 1987). However, these were used for research purposes, and as such, are not necessarily suitable for clinical use. These kinds of instrument are often rather long and detailed and would be too time-consuming to be used on a routine basis. Some also involve assessments involving visual analogue scales, which, as already mentioned, a small but significant proportion of patients find difficult to understand.

Realistically, it is better to focus on a small number of the more important aspects of patients' sleep in hospital settings. These include quality (how well they slept), quantity (how much sleep

Do you usually drink something before you go to sleep? Yes ☐   No ☐ What?
Do you usually eat something before you go to sleep?   Yes ☐   No ☐ What?
What else do you like to do before retiring to bed (if anything)?
How many pillows do you like?
What bedding do you prefer? (duvet, blankets, etc.)
What position do you like to go to sleep in?
Do you like to sleep with the window open?
Do you prefer to sleep with a light on or off?
Do you need absolute quiet in order to sleep?
Do you prefer your bedroom to be warm or cold in order to sleep?

Figure 5.8   Questions for a brief assessment of patients' sleep routine and preferences.

they had), and causes of disturbance, all of which can be noted in the Kardex and compared with their reported norms in their admission assessment. Problems may then be identified and action taken.

CONCLUSIONS

There are many different ways of assessing the various physiological and psychological changes occurring in association with sleep, as well as of making subjective assessments of sleep quality. When deciding on which method to use, first, and most importantly, the reason for monitoring sleep must be defined clearly. Is it because a hospital-based nurse wants to ensure that the ward environment is causing as little disruption to sleep as possible? Or because a community nurse wants to check whether a chronically tired client can benefit from advice only, or needs other kinds of help? Is it the quantity or the quality of sleep which is important?

The relevant aspects of sleep should be assessed using the methods most appropriate to the problem. Clearly a method which is convenient but which does not produce appropriate information is not worth using. Secondly, the cost of equipment and inconvenience to the patient should be considered. Many objective assessments (such as EEG recordings) necessitate the use of expensive equipment to which the majority of nurses would be unable to gain access and some patients might find such monitoring anxiety-provoking, restrictive or uncomfortable. While these approaches may be necessary for some kinds of research, they are not recommended for use in clinical practice.

Finally, individual patient factors pertinent to the chosen method should be considered. For example, patients with cataracts or arthritic fingers would not be able to complete a self-administered questionnaire, even if in theory it was the best way of gathering the data. Similar problems could be encountered when using subjective rating or visual analogue scales. These methods would be of little use for those with visual impairments or poor literacy. Similarly, an interview might not be possible with a deaf person.

The reason for assessing sleep should be defined as clearly as possible in order that an appropriate method of assessment may be used to provide valid and reliable results; the practicalities of using that method should be taken into account, and finally, variables such as age, and physical and psychological health should be considered when interpreting the results.

REFERENCES

Adam K, Oswald I 1984 Sleep helps healing. British Medical Journal 289: 1400–1401

Adam K, Tomeny M, Oswald I 1986 Physiological and psychological differences between good and poor sleepers. Journal of Psychiatric Research 20(4): 301–316

Aurell J, Elmqvist D 1985 Sleep in the surgical intensive care unit: continuous polygraphic recording of sleep in nine patients receiving postoperative care. British Medical Journal 290: 1029–1032

Bond A, Lader M 1974 The use of analogue scales in rating subjective feelings. British Journal of Medical Psychology 47: 211–218

Borkovec T D, Lane T W Van Oot PA 1981 Phenomenology of sleep among insomniacs and good sleepers: Wakefulness experience when cortically asleep. Journal of Abnormal Psychology 90(6): 607–609

Carskadon M, Dement W C 1979 Sleep tendency during extension of nocturnal sleep. Sleep Research 8: 147

Carskadon M, Dement W C, Mitler M M, Guilleminault C, Zarcone V P,
Spiegel R 1976 Self-reports versus sleep laboratory findings in 122 drug free
subjects with complaints of chronic insomnia. American Journal of Psychiatry
133: 1382–1388

Closs S J 1992 Surgical patients' experiences of sleep, night-time pain and
analgesic provision. PhD thesis, University of Edinburgh

Dodds E J 1980 Slept well? A study of ward activity and nurse–patient
interaction at night. MSc thesis, University of Surrey, Guildford

Edwards G B, Schuring L M 1993 Pilot study: validating staff nurses'
observations of sleep and wake states among critically ill patients, using
polysomnography. American Journal of Critical Care 2(2): 125–131

Edéll-Gustafsson U, Aren C, Hamrin E, Hetta J 1994 Nurses' notes on sleep
patterns in patients undergoing coronary artery bypass surgery:
a retrospective evaluation of patient records. Journal of Advanced Nursing
20: 331–336

Ehnfors M, Smedby B 1993 Nursing care as documented in patient records.
Scandinavian Journal of Caring Sciences 7(4): 209–220

Ellis B W, Johns M W, Lancaster R, Raptopoulos P, Angelopoulos N, Priest R G
1981 The St. Mary's Hospital Sleep Questionnaire: a study of reliability. Sleep
4(1): 93–97

Espie C A 1991 The psychological treatment of insomnia. Wiley, Chichester

Espie C A, Monk E, Hood E, Lindsay W R 1988 Establishing clinical criteria for
the treatment of chronic insomnia: a comparison of insomniac and control
populations. Health Bulletin 46(6): 318–326

Fontaine D K 1989 Measurement of nocturnal sleep patterns in trauma patients.
Heart and Lung 18(4): 402–410

Frankel B L, Course R D, Buchbinder R, Snyder F 1976 Recorded and reported
sleep in chronic insomnia. Archives of General Psychiatry 33: 615–623

Georgopolous B S, Jackson M 1970 Nursing Kardex behaviour in an
experimental study of patient units with and without clinical nurse
specialists. Nursing Research 19: 196–218

Hindmarch I, Parrott A C, Arenillas L A 1977 Repeated dose comparison of
dichloralphenazone, flunitrazepam and amylobarbitone sodium on some
aspects of sleep and early morning behaviour in normal subjects. British
Journal of Clinical Pharmacology 4: 229–233

Hoddes E, Dement W C, Zarcone V 1972 The history and use of the Stanford
Sleepiness Scale. (Abstract) Psychophysiology 9: 150

Johns M W 1991 A new method for measuring daytime sleepiness: the Epworth
Sleepiness Scale. Sleep 14(6): 540–545

Johns M W, Cornell B A, Masterton J P 1969 Monitoring sleep of hospital
patients by measurement of electrical resistance of skin. Journal of Applied
Physiology 27: 898–901

Kupfer D J, Wyatt R J, Snyder F 1970 Comparison between
electroencephalographic and systematic nursing observations of sleep in
psychiatric patients. Journal of Nervous and Mental Disorders 151: 361–368

Lacks P 1987 Behavioural treatment for persistent insomnia. Pergamon,
New York, pp 63–65

Lader M (ed) 1992 The medical management of insomnia in general practice.
Royal Society of Medicine Round Table Series 28, Royal Society of Medicine,
London

McClusky H Y et al 1991 Efficacy of behavioural versus triazolam treatment in
persistent sleep-onset insomnia. American Journal of Psychiatry 148: 121–125

Monroe L J (1967) Psychological and physiological differences between good and
poor sleepers. Journal of Abnormal Psychology 72: 255–264

Morgan K, Gledhill K 1991 Managing sleep and insomnia in the older person. Winslow Press, Bicester

Morin C M 1993 Insomnia: psychological assessment and management. Guilford Press, New York

National Medical Advisory Committee 1994 The management of anxiety and insomnia. HMSO, Edinburgh

Oswald I 1980 Sleep studies in clinical pharmacology. British Journal of Pharmacology 10: 317–326

Regestein Q R, Morris J 1987 Daily sleep patterns observed among institutionalized elderly residents. Journal of the American Geriatrics Society 35: 767–772

Rogers A E, Caruso C C, Aldrich M S 1993 Reliability of sleep diaries for assessment of sleep/wake patterns. Nursing Research 42(6): 368–372

Snyder-Halpern R, Verran J A 1987 Instrumentation to describe subjective sleep characteristics in healthy subjects. Research in Nursing and Health 10: 155–163

Tomeny M, Morgan K 1990 Management of insomnia in a primary care sleep clinic. Geriatric Medicine 20(6): 47–50

Webb W B 1965 Sleep characteristics of human subjects. Bulletin of the British Psychological Society 18: 1–10

Weiss B L, McPartland R L, Kupfer D L 1973 Once more: the inaccuracy of non-EEG estimates of sleep. American Journal of Psychiatry 130: 1282–1285

Williams R L, Karacan I, Hursch C J 1974 EEG of human sleep. John Wiley, New York, pp 51–64

Zealley A K, Aitken R C B 1969 Measurement of mood. Proceedings of the Royal Society of Medicine 62: 993–996

6

Sleep hygiene

Learning outcomes

Following assessment, the next step in managing a sleep problem is to identify and modify those everyday habits and practices which antagonise sleep, and encourage those behaviours which promote sleep. Referred to as 'sleep hygiene', this approach provides the foundation for all subsequent treatment, and can sometimes deliver sufficient improvement in sleep quality to make additional therapy unnecessary. Building on, and extending, some of the information already considered in Chapter 3, this chapter focuses on modifying factors known to disrupt sleep, and encouraging factors known to promote sleep. On completing this chapter you should be able to:

- name three common practices which may influence sleep quality
- explain the relevance of 'threshold effects' in sleep-related practices
- distinguish between ideal and optimal behavioural change
- negotiate a bed-time contract for use in clinical situations.

INTRODUCTION

Having assessed the dimensions of the presenting (or suspected) sleep problem it is now appropriate to take a closer look at the patient's general habits and behaviours (this can be done during the 10- to 14-day period when the first serial ratings are accumulating, or after the first sleep assessment interview). Collectively, this component of treatment, and the health education which usually accompanies it, is referred to as 'sleep hygiene'. The aim of sleep hygiene is twofold. First, to minimise the impact of disruptive factors on poor sleep and to optimise conditions for improving sleep quality. And second, to provide the basis for future prevention after the main problem responds to treatment.

What is sleep hygiene?

As already suggested in Chapter 3, the clinical and research literature has established clear links between aspects of lifestyle (e.g. diet, exercise, sleeping habits, etc.) and sleep quality. For example, sleep quality has been associated with caffeine consumption (Karacan et al 1976, Morgan et al 1989), unaccustomed night-time food-drinks (Adam 1980), pre-sleep alcohol use (see Zarcone 1994), levels of daytime stimulation (Horne & Minard 1985), cigarette smoking (Soldatos et al 1980), body weight (Adam 1987) and, among elderly people, excessive daytime napping (Ancoli-Israel et al 1989).

Improvements in sleep hygiene, on the other hand, have been associated with significant and sustained improvements in sleep quality, particularly when combined with psychological therapies (see Lacks 1987, Schoicket et al 1988). While sleep hygiene measures may not always be associated with significant improvements in sleep quality (see Espie 1991 for review), they provide a logical stage in the development of treatment, and should not be overlooked. Certainly, regularising daytime and night-time activities, optimising daytime stimulation, minimising daytime naps, and maximising the psychological association between the bedroom and sleep all make a significant contribution to the maintenance of satisfactory sleep–wake cycles.

Diet, activity and drug use

Broadly, the lifestyle issues mentioned above fall into the three major categories of: diet; activity; and drug use. This section looks briefly at the evidence base for advice relating to some of the more common practices and assumptions which affect sleep. (Aspects of all three categories were also discussed in Ch. 3.)

Diet and bedtime drinks

For many people, a drink at bedtime forms an intrinsic part of their pre-sleep behaviour, and many beverages have earned a reputation for promoting sleep. Nevertheless, it may become necessary to reconsider even well-established personal habits. If, for example, nocturia has become a problem in an older patient (i.e. if the associated sleep disturbance has become a source of distress and daytime sleepiness), bedtime drinking is probably best avoided altogether. If, on the other hand, a bedtime drink is considered desirable, then it should be noted that caffeinated drinks, (such as tea, coffee, cocoa, and many soft drinks) possess both stimulant and diuretic properties and may not be entirely suitable for those with fragile sleep.

Malted milk drinks like Ovaltine and Horlicks have long been associated with 'good' sleep. While the research evidence suggests that this reputation is not entirely unfounded, it also suggests that the value of these drinks depends very much upon the dietary habits of the individuals (a point made in Ch. 3). In electroencephalogram (EEG) laboratory studies it was found that among those accustomed to foods taken late at night, Horlicks was associated with better sleep (which, in this case, meant that sleep was longer and less broken). Conversely, among those unaccustomed to late night food, Horlicks at bedtime was associated with shorter, more broken sleep relative to that recorded on non-Horlicks nights (Adam 1980). Such findings also help to emphasise the principle that the maintenance of regular personal habits can optimise sleep quality (providing, of course, those personal habits are not in themselves detrimental to sleep).

Weight change and sleep. Changes in body weight can also significantly affect quality of sleep. In studies of obese subjects losing weight, for example, significant weight loss was found to be associated with reduced total sleep, and early morning awakening. Conversely, weight gain in those individuals with a history of anorexia nervosa was associated with improved sleep and later awakening. In subsequent studies of different patient groups, the point illustrated by these rather extreme examples has been confirmed – loss of weight can result in loss of sleep (see Crisp 1980 for review).

Activity and exercise

While it might seem intuitively plausible that exercise facilitates sound sleep, research evidence for such a relationship is far from clear cut. In an extensive review of over 90 theoretical papers and experimental studies concerned with the effects of exercise upon sleep, Horne (1980) concluded that non-athletes 'appear to show little, if any, sleep EEG effects following daytime exercise'. Among highly-trained athletes, however, an increase in slow wave sleep has been observed on those nights which followed vigorous daily training sessions. During sleep, EEG slow waves are associated with certain restorative processes, and it is likely that a change in this sleep stage is mediated by the body's need for restoration after the physiological wear and tear of training. Given that the relationship between such changes (i.e. increases in slow waves) and subjective sleep quality remains unclear, the apparent benefits to sleep of intense exercise are of little practical relevance to most people. There are, however, other ways in which exercise can influence sleep apart from its physiological cost.

Many forms of moderate exercise can engender feelings which are themselves conductive to sleep, like tranquillity, personal satisfaction and well-being, and even sleepiness. Evidence that general daytime stimulation can facilitate sleep is provided by Horne & Minard (1985). In a group of nine healthy young female students, sleep EEGs were recorded after 2 'baseline' days of routine academic work in the library or laboratory, and after an 'experimental' day characterised by 'interest, variety and novelty', during which the student was taken to the zoo, an amusement park, and finally to the cinema in several cross-country car journeys. After the experimental day, volunteers were subjectively sleepier (as measured by a sleep questionnaire), fell asleep more rapidly, and showed longer periods of slow wave sleep than after the baseline days. Thus, whether perceived as exercise or not, activities which result in both mental and physical stimulation have implications for improved sleep quality.

Drug use and sleep

A discussion of drug effects on sleep is provided in Chapter 3. In addition to social drugs like caffeine and alcohol, it should be remembered that some therapeutic drugs can also affect (and sometimes seriously affect) sleep quality. In some patients, such a response may be idiosyncratic, such that substituting a given product for one generically similar may be beneficial. An important nursing consideration here is to become familiar with the possible impact of new and established therapeutics on sleep and wakefulness.

Environmental factors

The sleep hygiene factors considered so far have, for the most part, been centred on the patient's behaviour. Two additional factors, both with implications for sleep quality, concern elements in the patient's environment: the bed partner, and the bedroom.

The bed partner

The presence of a bed partner, or even other persons within the same household can, it appears, have considerable implications for sleep continuity and quality. In an extensive field study of the effects of aircraft noise on the sleep of people living near Heathrow Airport, London, for example, Horne et al (1994) found that the behaviour of bed partners and others living in the household appeared to be a more influential factor than ageing in determining intrasleep arousals (as measured using actigraphy – wrist-worn activity monitors). Perhaps, then, sleeping arrangements may also be reconsidered where sleep difficulties become severe.

The sleep environment

In the light of the research findings discussed in Chapter 3, three questions seem especially pertinent when assessing the sleep environment, which may not be a bedroom. First, is the sleep environment warm enough? Second, is the sleep environment quiet enough? As increasing age is associated with a progressive reduction in the auditory awakening threshold, the quietest possible environment is to be recommended. Previously preferred bedrooms in the front of the house overlooking the street, for example, might wisely be vacated for a quieter back bedroom. Finally, is the bed itself sufficiently comfortable? Worn bedsprings and saggy mattresses can be detrimental to sound sleep, and can lead to joint aches and pains during the daytime.

OFFERING SLEEP HYGIENE

Advice is useless if the recipients do not see a need to cooperate, or if they feel it does not apply to them. This introduces the need both to *assess* the patient's habits and practices before offering advice, and to *introduce* the advice with a brief, positive explanation. The first of these points is self-explanatory. Admonishing non-smokers to stop smoking, or those who already avoid caffeine to drink less tea, will do little for the credibility of the adviser or the advice. (Indeed, the research evidence suggests that poor sleepers tend to have a better knowledge of sleep hygiene matters than good sleepers; see Lacks & Rotert 1986.) As for the second point, it is helpful to begin by pointing out to the patient, quite simply, that sleep hygiene approaches are clinically effective, and common sense. Once again, it should be explained that the measures suggested are intended to improve sleep quality, and not to cure insomnia. To avoid unnecessary disappointment, it should also be made clear that these measures: (a) are unlikely to improve sleep quality if practised only episodically, and (b) are unlikely to produce benefits within the first 1–2 weeks. Finally, do not ask for too much. The needs of the patient must always be considered, with sometimes optimal rather than ideal changes agreed. On the other hand, be careful not to overcompromise and simply encourage minor and clinically useless changes in personal behaviours.

Threshold effects

The issue of resistance from patients to their involvement in sleep management was addressed in Chapter 4 (it might be useful to re-read this section now). Keep in mind that one of the major attributes of effective hypnotic drugs, which have done so much to shape the culture of treatment in this area, is that they work passively, and require little from the patient. One consequence of this is that we are all unaccustomed to participating in treatment.

One special source of resistance among (particularly older) poor sleepers concerns the operation of threshold effects in physiological tolerance. Simply put, some poor sleepers are not easily convinced that a life-long habit or practice, previously accompanied by sound sleep, may be contributing to their current problem. Sensitivity to a number of 'sleep antagonists' (e.g. caffeine, noise, irregular hours) can change with age and personal circumstances. When sensitivity reaches a critical threshold, sleep is disturbed. It is helpful, therefore, if the operation of such threshold effects is explained. Certainly, a lifestyle characterised by irregular sleeping times, repeated episodes of sleep deprivation, and expectations of weekly 'recovery sleep' (a lifestyle captured in the metaphor 'burning the candle at both ends') is unlikely to be physiologically tolerated as sleep ages into its third and fourth decade.

Assessment

The sleep hygiene assessment can be performed as an extension of the initial sleep interview, though it will be better informed once sleep diaries or other serial assessments have accumulated. A list of possible targets for sleep hygiene advice is provided in the sleep hygiene checklist shown in Table 6.1. Information from sleep diaries and/or sleep questionnaires can also be used to identify the patients' typical sleep and bedtime patterns, and their personal expectations of sleep. If sleeping habits have clearly broken down (i.e. eccentric bedtimes, obvious lack of routine), or where time spent in bed is clearly excessive (as may happen among the retired, unemployed, or depressed), bedtimes and getting up times (specifically, times before which the patient cannot retire, and after which he or she cannot stay in bed) can be agreed in the form of a 'contract', an actual document containing the times agreed. (A suggested format for such a document is provided in Box 7.1 in the next chapter, p 111.)

Table 6.1   A sleep hygiene checklist

Question	Consider intervention if the answer is:
1. Does the patient have realistic expectations of sleep quality and quantity?	No
2. Does the patient maintain fairly regular habits (e.g. bedtimes, getting-up times, meal times)?	No
3. Could the patient's bedroom be quieter or more comfortable?	Yes
4. Does the patient drink caffeinated drinks close to bedtime or during the night?	Yes
5. Does the patient use alcohol as a sleep inducer?	Yes
6. Does the patient have an identifiable pre-sleep routine?	No
7. Does the patient nap habitually?	Yes
8. Is the patient usually tired on retiring?	No
9. Is the patient choosing when to go to bed?	No
10. Is the patient usually tired/sleepy during the day?	Yes
11. Is the patient taking any prescribed medicine with known disruptive effects on sleep?	Yes

The following summary extends the brief items presented in Table 6.1, and can serve as an interview structure.

Summary of sleep hygiene issues

• The patient's expectations of sleep may provide important insights into the origins of dissatisfaction with sleep. There is little research evidence to suggest, however, that unrealistic expectations are a major source of sleep complaints – at any age.

• Chronic poor sleep is frequently accompanied and exacerbated by a corruption of the circadian (24-hour) sleep–wake cycle. To restore and preserve an optimal 24-hour rhythm in sleep, regular times must be observed for meals, activity, going to bed, getting up and, if taken, naps. If necessary, contract bedtimes and getting up times.

• Improvements in the sleep environment can produce improvements in sleep quality.

• Sleep quality can be greatly affected by both alcohol and caffeine, and it is reasonable to focus special attention on these widely used social drugs. While caffeine can delay sleep onset, alcohol can, in certain quantities, disturb sleep in the latter part of the night. Certainly, among poor sleepers, caffeine ingestion should be minimal, while the use of alcohol as a sleep inducer is best avoided.

• Methodical pre-sleep routines (e.g. finish cocoa, television off, milk bottles out, cat in, brush teeth, etc.) serve as important behavioural signals for 'winding down' before bed and should be encouraged. Ritual and routine are the guardians of fragile sleep. (These points will be developed in the next chapter.)

• Weight loss, particularly severe weight loss, can be associated with reductions in sleep quality, and is a frequently overlooked cause of insomnia.

• It is widely supposed that certain milky drinks contribute to restful sleep. In fact, this is only partly true. If individuals are accustomed to taking milky drinks (or light snacks) close to bedtime, then their sleep might well be a little disturbed if they break this habit. If, on the other hand, people are unused to snacking late in the evening, then milk drinks or any other food taken at this time might actually disturb their sleep.

• In retirement, regularly scheduled naps can be refreshing and satisfying and are not in themselves a problem. However, napping can be particularly unhelpful if it results from boredom or exhaustion (whether among the retired, the unemployed, or the chronically ill). Under these circumstance it will probably have a detrimental impact on night-time sleep.

• Exercise close to bedtime can produce a state of arousal incompatible with sleep. Exercise, if taken, is probably best avoided in the late evening. The only exception to this is sexual activity which, for a variety of reasons, can actually promote sleep.

• Prescribed medicines should not be overlooked as a possible cause of sleep problems. In particular, some antihypertensives (methyldopa, beta-blockers) can produce sleeplessness and nightmares. Diuretics, too, can remain active at night, and can also cause night-time cramps.

Monitoring

As with other components of treatment, the impact of sleep hygiene measures can be monitored using the serial assessment methods already discussed. Such feedback will indicate the success of, or the need to modify the advice given. It will also provide the signal to develop therapy further. If treatment is to be developed, then existing sleep hygiene measures should be retained.

REFERENCES

Adam K 1980 Dietary habits and sleep after bedtime food drinks. Sleep 3: 47–58
Adam K 1987 Total and percentage REM sleep correlate with body weight in 36 middle-aged people. Sleep 10: 69–77
Ancoli-Israel S, Parker L, Sinaee R, Fell R L, Kripke D F 1989 Sleep fragmentation in patients from a nursing home. Journal of Gerontology: Medical Sciences 44: M18–21
Crisp A 1980 Sleep, activity, nutrition and mood. British Journal of Psychiatry 137: 1–7
Espie C A 1991 The psychological treatment of insomnia. Wiley, Chichester
Horne J A 1980 The effects of exercise upon sleep: a critical review. Biological Psychiatry 12: 241–290
Horne J A, Minard A 1985 Sleep and sleepiness following a behaviourally 'active' day. Ergonomics 28: 567–575
Horne J A, Pankhurst F L, Reyner L A, Hume K, Diamond I D 1994 A field study of sleep disturbance: effects of aircraft noise and other factors on 5,742 nights of actimetrically monitored sleep in a large subject sample. Sleep 17: 146–159
Karacan I, Thornby J I, Anch H et al 1976 The prevalence of sleep disturbance in a primarily urban Florida county. Social Science and Medicine 10: 239–244

Lacks P, Rotert M 1986 Knowledge and practice of sleep hygiene techniques in
    insomniacs and good sleepers. Behaviour Research and Therapy 24: 365–368
Lacks P 1987 Behavioral treatment for persistent insomnia. Pergamon, New York
Morgan K, Healey D W, Healey P J 1989 Factors influencing persistent subjective
    insomnia in old age: a follow-up study of good and poor sleepers aged
    65–74. Age and Ageing 18: 117–122
Schoicket S A, Bertelson A D, Lacks P 1988 Is sleep hygiene a sufficient treatment
    for sleep-maintenance insomnia. Behavior Therapy 19: 183–190
Soldatos C R, Kales J D, Scharf M B, Bixler E O, Kales A 1980 Cigarette smoking
    associated with sleep difficulty. Science 207: 551–552
Zarcone V P 1994 Sleep hygiene. In: Kryger M H, Roth T, Dement W C (eds)
    Principles and practice of sleep medicine, 2nd edn. W B Saunders,
    Philadelphia

7

Habits, learning and sleep: stimulus control treatment for insomnia

---

Learning outcomes

It was suggested in Chapter 4 (see Table 4.1, p. 64) that the optimal response to insomnia begins with simpler interventions and, if necessary, progresses through to the more complex therapies. Having assessed, and taken steps to improve sleep hygiene, it is now appropriate to consider how the patient's habits and personal routines may be affecting his or her sleep quality. This chapter introduces the theory and practice of stimulus control therapy as applied to insomnia. On completing this chapter you should be able to:

- describe the role of learning in the control of sleep onset
- describe circumstances under which the stimulus control of sleep onset may be reduced
- describe the possible role of classical conditioning in maintaining insomnia
- offer appropriate advice on whether reading in bed is a good thing, or a bad thing.

INTRODUCTION

What is stimulus control?

Many activities tend to occur in specific settings and under quite specific circumstances. Sleep, for example, tends to occur in bed, in bedrooms, at night; eating takes place at tables, and at specific times throughout the day. Over time, through the processes of learning or 'conditioning', these settings and circumstances become signals, and sometimes quite powerful signals, for the behaviours associated with them. Once this relationship is well established, the presence of these signals actually makes the behaviours associated with them much more likely. Lying down in bed, for example, can promote sleep, while sitting down to eat a meal can stimulate appetite. In psychological theory, a signal which sets the occasion for a particular behavioural response is called a 'discriminative stimulus', while the relationship which develops between the stimulus and the behavioural response it encourages is referred to as the 'stimulus control' of that behaviour. In chronic insomnia, however, where long periods in bed are increasingly associated with wakefulness, connections between these discriminative stimuli and sleep onset can be significantly weakened. As originally proposed by Bootzin (1972), this attenuation or loss of stimulus control can contribute to both the onset and maintenance of insomnia.

The process is not always passive. A person experiencing long periods of insomnia may actively encourage the weakening of stimulus control by engaging in a variety of non-sleep activities in the bedroom (e.g. eating, smoking, watching television, listening to the radio). Not only do such activities weaken the original associations between bedroom and sleep, they may actually convert what were stimuli for rest (i.e. aspects of the bedroom environment) into cues for arousal.

Types of learning

Stimulus control theory, therefore, emphasises that, while sleep itself is a biologically programmed behaviour, it is nevertheless greatly influenced by processes of learning. Psychology distinguishes between two kinds of learning or conditioning which are relevant here. (Useful descriptions of conditioning paradigms, and their application to nursing practice, can be found in Fisher (1990).) Operant (or instrumental) conditioning results from the selective reinforcement of previously emitted behaviour, making that behaviour more likely to recur. In the archetypal experiments of B F Skinner, for example, rats rewarded by food pellets immediately after they pressed a lever became much more likely to engage in lever pressing. Classical (or Pavlovian) conditioning, on the other hand, results from the pairing of *conditioned* and *unconditioned* stimuli (in Pavlov's classic experiments, a bell and the presentation of food, respectively) such that the conditioned stimulus alone comes to elicit the now conditioned response (canine salivation in Pavlov's experiments). As a behaviour reinforced by sleep itself, efficient sleep *onset* (and the stimuli associated with it) provides an example of *operant* learning. However, through the repeated pairing of bedroom cues with the frustrations and anxieties of sleeplessness, these same stimuli can now, through the mechanisms of *classical* conditioning, become conditioned stimuli for negative emotional responses (frustration, anger, irritation) which antagonise and sustain episodes of insomnia. The simple aim of stimulus control treatment, therefore, is to maximise the sleep promoting properties of the bedroom environment (Bootzin & Nicassio 1978, Bootzin et al 1991). The underlying logic of treatment is that what has been learned, and un-learned (or, in the terminology of learning theory, *extinguished*), can be relearned. In practice this means systematically re-establishing or strengthening links between the sleep environment and sleep.

Stimulus control and the origins of insomnia

In addition to providing a rational theoretical basis for treatment, these operant and classical conditioning processes have important implications for understanding both the nature and the origins of some chronic insomnias. In particular, they draw attention to the possibility that factors which can *cause* a sleep problem may be unrelated to factors which *maintain* a sleep problem (a process summarised in Fig. 7.1). Consider the following case example.

Mr F's insomnia

Mr F fractured his humerus while playing rugby. Otherwise fit, and never a poor sleeper, Mr F experienced considerable sleeplessness in the weeks following the surgery to pin his broken bone. Even after the constant pain had resolved, the limitations on his sleeping position continued to antagonise his sleep. Irritated with his insomnia, Mr F adapted to his new circumstances by preparing for episodes of wakefulness. He took the newspaper, and light snacks, into his bedroom, and began listening to his radio when awake at night (just for company). Increasingly,

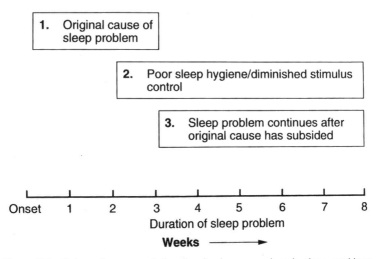

Figure 7.1 Schematic representation showing how poor sleep hygiene, and loss of stimulus control can maintain a sleep problem after the original cause has ceased to play a part. (1) The impact of direct causal factors (pain, occupational stress, etc.) may last only for a matter of weeks. (2) Personal responses to this sleeplessness may be characterised by poor sleep hygiene, and result in diminished stimulus control. (3) Psychological and sleep hygiene factors can now maintain the insomnia, even though the original cause has subsided.

however, he found it more and more difficult to get to sleep. Since he was off work with his injury and somewhat limited in his activities, he also became bored during the day. Boredom, coupled with his daytime sleepiness, lead to naps in front of the afternoon television. As a result, he was less sleepy when he went to bed, and consequently less inclined to fall asleep. After 4 weeks, he returned to work. His operative scars had healed, his arm was pain-free, and the range of movement in the injured limb was close to his pre-injury level. But he had acquired a disturbing sleep problem.

Perhaps Mr F had always had vulnerable sleep (see Ch. 2), and his injury, together with his subsequent behaviour, unmasked this predisposition (after all, not everyone with an injury develops a sleep problem). Whatever the case, assessment of Mr F's sleeping habits, combined with his recent sleep and clinical history, clearly identified loss of stimulus control as a likely contributing factor to maintenance of the present sleep problem. The treatment plan, therefore, aimed to restore the association between bedroom and sleep which had been lost during Mr F's rehabilitation.

Stimulus control and sleep hygiene

With an emphasis on sleep-related habits, and the promotion of optimal circumstances to induce sleep, stimulus control procedures are a natural extension of (and, to some extent, overlap with) the sleep hygiene procedures described in the previous chapter. Certainly, given the connections between them, it is reasonable at assessment to examine both sleep hygiene and stimulus control issues, and identify a common set of treatment goals. It is, nevertheless, useful to keep these approaches conceptually separate. Sleep hygiene advice is based upon assumed, usually physiological (e.g. the stimulant properties of drugs; the arousing consequences of exercise) connections between certain practices and sleep onset and continuity. Stimulus control procedures, on the other hand, are based upon rules derived from experimental studies of learning.

Treatment outcomes

In recent years, stimulus control procedures have emerged as one of the most successful psychological methods for treating insomnia (Lacks & Morin 1992, Morin et al 1994). In addition to providing benefits in the shorter term (1–3 months), these procedures have also been associated with high levels of patient adherence, and sustained therapeutic benefits (Lacks & Morin 1992, Morin et al 1994). Given the increasing likelihood of insomnia in later life, it is also relevant to note that stimulus control treatments have been found effective in the management of late-life insomnias (e.g. Morin & Azrin 1988, Puder et al 1983). Nevertheless, some of the standard stimulus control instructions (leaving the bedroom in the night, for example) may not be appropriate for all elderly patients (see below).

STIMULUS CONTROL TREATMENT FOR INSOMNIA

As already emphasised, the aim of stimulus control treatment is to help the patient relearn and benefit from pre-insomnia associations between sleep and the sleep environment. This relearning process has two components: (a) maximising the opportunity to associate the bed and bedroom with rest and sleep; and (b) minimising the opportunity to associate the bedroom with any sleep-incompatible behaviours. In general, then, the emphasis is on reducing to a minimum the amount time spent *awake* in bed.

Stimulus control and sleep restriction therapy

Where insomnia is accompanied by excessive amounts of time spent in bed (excessive, that is, relative to the amount of actual sleep achieved), sleep restriction therapy has been associated with marked improvements. As a formal therapy, sleep restriction involves an agreement with patients to reduce their time in bed so that it matches their estimated time asleep. Thus, if a patient spends 9 hours in bed but, on average, achieves only 7 hours of sleep, then 7 hours in bed would at first be recommended (see Spielman et al 1987). The recommended time in bed can then be reviewed weekly and varied according to the average sleep efficiency index (calculated as: (Total sleep time ÷ Time in bed) × 100) for the preceding week. Time in bed can be increased by 15 minutes if the average sleep for the previous week (as measured by sleep diaries) exceeds 90%, or decreased by the same amount if average sleep efficiency falls below 85% (Spielman et al 1987). In practice, recommendations to spend less than, say, 4 hours in bed are likely to meet with resistance from the patient (however low the sleep efficiency index), so a lower limit of approximately 4–5 hours has been suggested (Morin 1993). Like sleep hygiene, the sleep restriction approach to therapy fits well with stimulus control procedures, and may be included in an overall therapeutic 'package'. The stimulus control approach to insomnia outlined below, therefore, departs slightly from that suggested by Bootzin et al (1991) in that it includes an implicit, though flexible, sleep restriction component (setting the bed-time and getting-up time). It should be emphasised, however, that under some circumstances sleep restriction alone can provide an effective therapy for insomnia, and has been successfully used among hospital inpatients (Morin et al 1990).

Stimulus control: assessment and monitoring

As suggested above, the assessment of sleep hygiene (Ch. 6), and the assessment of factors influencing stimulus control can usefully be conducted together, since both issues can overlap. Information from the initial sleep assessment (Ch. 5) and accumulated daily sleep diaries can first be used to align patients' estimated time in bed with their estimated total sleep time. One way to achieve this is to estimate and suggest the amount of sleep per night that patients can reasonably expect (this may well be a compromise between what they would like, and what they actually get). For example, if a patient appears to expect 7–8 hours' sleep per night, but the sleep diaries clearly indicate an average of 5–6 hours' sleep per night, it is reasonable to encourage a lower and more realistic expectation. Next, negotiate with patients a time of going to bed and getting up sufficient for them to accumulate this agreed amount of sleep (include a reasonable time to fall asleep, say 15–20 minutes). In the early stages of treatment the agreed bedtime can be interpreted as a time *before which* the patient will not go to bed. Thus, if patients do not feel sleepy at the agreed time, they may go to bed later (but, of course, they must be out of bed by the agreed getting-up time in the morning). Record the agreed times on a patient information sheet similar to that shown in Box 7.1. Progress should be reviewed weekly for the first 4 weeks. As sleep efficiency improves, time in bed may be extended, with adjustments made to bedtimes and getting-up times.

Box 7.1 Stimulus control treatment for insomnia: patient information sheet and contract

The treatment recommended for your sleep problem is called stimulus control therapy. This is a very effective treatment for problems like yours, but it will only work if you follow the advice given.

General advice
1. The time we have agreed for your going to bed at night is _____ (time)
2. The time we have agreed for your getting up in the morning is _____ (time)
3. During treatment please observe the agreed rules.

At first this treatment may make you a little sleepy during the day. It may be helpful, therefore, if you tell your family and friends about your treatment plan, and its possible effects. In time, improvements in your sleep will actually make you feel more alert.

Expectations and recovery sleep

In discussing sleep expectations with patients, the following point may be helpful. People suffering from chronic insomnia frequently experience considerable night-to-night variations in their total sleep time, with the tiredness which accumulates from several poor nights eventually resulting in a single, atypical, night of relatively unbroken sleep. This situation is similar to that seen in laboratory studies of partial or total sleep deprivation, where the accumulated sleep 'debt' is followed by a 'recovery sleep' characterised by long periods of stage 4 and REM (see Horne 1988). Among chronic insomnia sufferers it is possible that such recovery sleep may occasionally be interpreted as their 'normal' sleep, and offered as a personal goal. However, since recovery sleep requires antecedent sleep deprivation, it is really part of the problem, and should be explained as such.

The rules of stimulus control treatment

Having agreed bedtimes (or times before which the individual cannot go to bed) and getting-up times, the patient should now be asked to observe the rules given in Box 7.2 (these are based on the proposals of Bootzin & Nicassio (1978), and Bootzin et al (1991)). It is essential that each rule is clearly understood. In presenting stimulus control procedures, therefore, the rationale underlying each rule should be explained to, and the rule itself discussed with the patient. Satisfy yourself that the patient is both willing and able to comply with the instructions. Where adherence is unlikely (for example some elderly patients may not wish to leave their bedrooms for long periods during the night) a compromise may be introduced (such as sitting beside the bed).

Box 7.2　Rules for stimulus control management

1. Do not go to bed before the agreed time.
2. Go to bed only when tired, and lie down with the intention of going to sleep.
3. If you do not fall asleep within 20 minutes,* get up, go to another room, and engage in some reasonably quiet and relaxing activity.
4. Do not use the bedroom for any activity other than sleeping (sexual activity is the only exception here). In particular, avoid reading, eating, smoking, listening to the radio or watching television in your bedroom).
5. If, having returned to bed, you do not fall asleep within 20 minutes,* observe rule 3.
6. Set your alarm clock for the agreed getting-up time, and get up at that time each morning. Never lie in, even if you feel tired in the morning.
7. Avoid all daytime napping (this includes falling asleep in a chair before going to bed).

*Flexibility may be appropriate here; older patients may require more time.

Stimulus control procedures, combined with appropriate adjustments in sleep hygiene, can be effective within 3–4 weeks if practised appropriately (Lacks 1987). Monitoring of sleep (using sleep diaries or daily records) should continue throughout this period, and follow-up sessions (to discuss progress and encourage adherence) are advisable. The effort required of the patient, however, should not be underestimated. Some patients will find the procedures difficult, and will need particular encouragement and support. It is also possible that some aspects of treatment will give more concern than others, and adjustments may be necessary (for example, variations in bedtimes or getting-up times). Allow several weeks for sleep to settle down under the new regime before proceeding with further management initiatives.

Finally, it should be noted that people who do *not* complain of insomnia may find some of the proscribed activities listed above as both pleasant and important components of their own sleep routines. Reading in bed, for example, can provide individuals with the necessary escape, relaxation, and comfort to trigger restful and satisfying sleep. Clearly, then, it is not the practice of reading (or listening to the radio, or watching television) per se which promotes insomnia, but rather the repeated association of these behaviours with unsuccessful attempts to get to sleep. Where these activities are associated with good sleep quality, they are best maintained.

SLEEP HYGIENE AND STIMULUS CONTROL TREATMENT: A CASE STUDY

The following case study describes an actual patient who was successfully treated with stimulus control procedures.

Background

Mr G was a 67-year-old married man with a 30-year history of insomnia and hypnotic drug use. He had retired at 65, much of his working life having been spent as a shift-worker in the post office. Though mildly hypertensive (for which he took beta-blockers), he was otherwise healthy. Having weaned himself off benzodiazepines, and been hypnotic drug-free for over 6 months, he had returned to his general practitioner complaining of very long sleep latencies (up to 2 hours) and unrefreshing sleep. He had requested hypnotics, but was offered instead a referral to a specialist clinical psychology service (Tomeny & Morgan 1990), which he accepted.

Presentation

For a period of 1 week prior to his appointment Mr G completed sleep diaries which were sent to him with his appointment letter. He was then assessed using a sleep assessment questionnaire (Fig. 5.1, p. 76) and a sleep hygiene checklist (Table 6.1, p. 101), in addition to a clinical interview which included those issues covered in the Lacks' (1987) sleep questionnaire (Fig. 5.2, p. 78).

From these assessments it was clear that Mr G had problems both with his sleep hygiene and in the stimulus control of his sleep. A particular, rather obsessional man, Mr G spent much of his day in his garden, or in his allotment (where he grew vegetables). He would go indoors for his supper in the evening between 5–7 p.m. (depending on the season). However, before sitting down to eat, he would first take a bath after which, not wanting to put on clean clothes 'just for a couple of hours', he dressed in his pyjamas.

Habitually, he would retire to bed (alone) at about 10 p.m. 'Knowing' he would not fall asleep straight away, he would take a newspaper or gardening magazine to read for a while. Mrs G would join her husband at about 11 p.m., usually taking him a cup of tea. After settling down, Mr G was frequently restless and rarely (from both his diaries and recollection) fell asleep before 1 a.m. In an attempt to compensate for lost sleep, Mr G would sleep in well after his wife had got up, and frequently had his morning tea in bed. In his sleep diaries, Mr G recorded sleep onset latencies of up to 120 minutes; his time in bed ranged from 8–10 hours, while his total sleep time rarely exceeded 6 hours per night.

Conclusions

Mr G's long history of insomnia was certainly exacerbated, or perhaps even caused, by his shift work. One legacy of this was that his expectations of satisfactory sleep were extremely low. Clearly, both Mr and Mrs G had reconciled themselves to Mr G's insomnia, and had created a domestic routine around the problem. This routine, however, was characterised by examples of poor sleep hygiene (going to bed when not tired, drinking tea too close to the sleep period), and behaviours antagonistic to optimal stimulus control (e.g. excessive periods awake in bed; regular engagement in non-sleep activities in the bedroom). Both provided targets for therapy.

Treatment

The following regime was discussed and agreed with Mr G. Following his bath, he would dress in day-clothes (pyjamas should be a cue for sleeping). He would not go to bed before 11.30 p.m., and would not drink tea or coffee after 8 p.m. He would also observe the stimulus control rules, getting up at 6 a.m. (even at weekends). Since his initial complaint had emphasised extended sleep onset latencies and unrefreshing sleep, it was also agreed that these characteristics would provide the focus for outcome measurement.

Outcome

Mr G responded well to the attention and concern of the therapist, and was personally encouraged by the small improvements which initially accompanied treatment. Persevering, both his sleep latency, and his sleep quality steadily improved over the treatment period. These improvements were maintained at 3- and 6-month follow-up. Averaged weekly scores from Mr G's sleep diaries are shown in Figure 7.2.

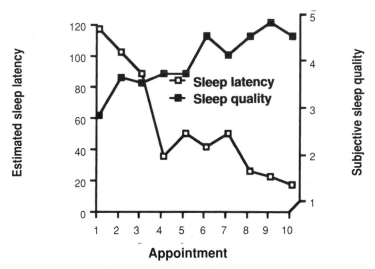

Figure 7.2   Averaged weekly sleep diary ratings of sleep latency (left vertical axis) and sleep quality (right vertical axis) for a 67-year-old man observing stimulus control procedures for insomnia. Improvements were maintained at 3- and 6-month follow-ups.

SUMMARY

Stimulus control procedures aim to promote sleep by strengthening the links between environmental cues for sleep, and sleep onset. These procedures complement those of sleep hygiene and sleep restriction, and can produce positive and lasting benefits after 3–4 weeks. Outcomes can be effectively monitored using sleep diaries.

REFERENCES

Bootzin R R 1972 Stimulus control treatment for insomnia. Proceedings of the American Psychological Association 7: 395–396
Bootzin R R, Nicassio P M 1978 Behavioral treatments for insomnia. In: Hersen M, Eisler R, Miller P (eds) Progress in behavior modification. Academic Press, New York, vol 6
Bootzin R R, Epstein D, Wood J M 1991 Stimulus control instructions. In: Hauri P (ed) Case studies in insomnia. Plenum Press, New York
Fisher E E 1990 Behavioural sciences for nurses: towards project 2000. Duckworth, London, pp 150–160
Horne J 1988 Why we sleep. The functions of sleep in humans and other mammals. Oxford University Press, Oxford
Lacks P 1987 Behavioral treatment of insomnia. Pergamon, New York
Lacks P, Morin C M 1992 Recent advances in the assessment and treatment of insomnia. Journal of Consulting and Clinical Psychology 60: 586–594
Morin C M 1993 Insomnia – psychological assessment and management. The Guilford Press, New York
Morin C M, Azrin N H 1988 Behavioral and cognitive treatments of geriatric insomnia. Journal of Consulting and Clinical Psychology 56: 748–753
Morin C M, Kowatch R A, O'Shanick G 1990 Sleep restriction for the inpatient treatment of insomnia. Sleep 13: 183–186
Morin C M, Culbert J P, Schwartz S M 1994 Nonpharmacological interventions for insomnia: a meta-analysis of treatment efficacy. American Journal of Psychiatry 151: 1172–1180
Puder R, Lacks P, Bertelson A D, Storandt M 1983 Short-term stimulus control treatment of insomnia in older adults. Behavior Therapy 14: 424–429
Spielman A J, Saskin P, Thorpy M J 1987 Treatment of chronic insomnia by restriction of time in bed. Sleep 10: 45–56
Tomeny M, Morgan K 1990 Management of insomnia in a primary care sleep clinic. Geriatric Medicine 20(6): 47–50

8

Tension and sleep: relaxation treatments for insomnia

Learning outcomes

The sleep hygiene and stimulus control procedures described in the previous two chapters make implicit assumptions about the underlying causes of insomnia: sleep antagonistic practices and maladaptive sleep habits respectively. The treatment approaches described in the next two chapters deal with the likely contribution of physical (autonomic) and cognitive (mental) arousal to insomnia. On completing this chapter you should be able to:

- discriminate between physiological and cognitive arousal
- recognise the value of relaxation in dealing with some types of insomnia
- describe two different relaxation procedures.

INTRODUCTION

Physiological arousal and sleep

One of the earliest theories guiding the psychological management of sleep proposed that insomnia was principally mediated by physiological (specifically autonomic) arousal, and that those with a predisposition to sleep poorly were more autonomically 'active' than those who generally slept well. This 'physiological hyperarousal' theory was supported by the seminal research of Monroe (1967), who assessed selected psychological and physiological characteristics of self-described 'good' and 'poor' sleepers.

117

When compared with the good sleepers, those who described their usual sleep as poor actually slept less (according to electroencephalogram (EEG) criteria), were more restless during sleep, had higher body temperatures, and tended to have a faster pulse-rate. While subsequent studies have failed to find such clear-cut differences between good and poor sleepers (see Borkovec 1982, Lacks 1987 for reviews), evidence of psychological and physiological differences between those who sleep well and those who do not continue to accrue (e.g. Adam et al 1986; see also Ch. 2). Following Monroe's study, the technique of progressive relaxation, first described by Jacobson (1929) and widely used in psychological therapy at that time, appeared to provide a means for reducing autonomic activity and thereby treating insomnia.

Jacobson's method of progressive relaxation (also referred to as progressive muscle relaxation or PMR) aims not only to relax tense muscles but also to improve subjective awareness of this relaxation. The technique has subsequently been modified by Bernstein & Borkovec (1973), whose procedures remain widely used. These revised and abbreviated procedures place even more emphasis on amplifying the somatic experience of relaxation. Thus, subjects (who are lying or sitting in a comfortable position and in a suitably quiet environment) are required first to tense specific muscle groups, and then to release all tension, allowing the structures supported by those muscles to become limp and heavy. This tension–release cycle can last up to 50 seconds (5–7 seconds of tension followed by about 45 seconds of release) for each muscle group, and is applied progressively to the muscle groups of limbs, trunk, and even the face (see Box 8.1). The procedure can result in significant reductions in heart rate and blood-pressure.

While there is now a substantial literature indicating that progressive relaxation can be of benefit in the treatment of sleep onset insomnia (see Espie 1991 for review), it is also clear that the procedures may work for reasons other than those originally assumed. A number of studies have reported significant reductions in sleep onset latency, obtained with progressive relaxation procedures, without reductions in autonomic activity (see Borkovec 1982). This mismatch between theory and therapy clearly indicates that other factors, beyond physiological arousal, are mediating both insomnia itself, and the effectiveness of progressive relaxation. As regards the efficacy of treatment, one strong candidate here is *cognitive* arousal. While autonomic arousal

---

Box 8.1   Progressive relaxation training: proposed sequence of muscle groups for tension/relaxation (proposed method of tensing)

1. Dominant hand/forearm (making a fist/pushing the palm down against the bed/arm of a chair)*
2. Dominant biceps (pushing the elbow down against the arm of a chair with hand relaxed)
3. Non-dominant hand/forearm
4. Non-dominant biceps
5. Forehead, upper cheeks and nose (furrow brow; tighten cheeks; wrinkle nose)
6. Lower cheeks and jaws (clenching the teeth, draw back the corners of the mouth)
7. Neck and throat (pull the chin down towards the sternum, and push head back against the chair)
8. Chest, shoulders and upper back (draw the shoulders back)
9. Abdomen (tighten the abdominal muscles, making them hard)
10. Dominant thigh (contract the knee flexors and extensors together)
11. Dominant calf (pull the foot up, towards the face)
12. Dominant foot (point the foot away from the face)
13. Non-dominant thigh
14. Non-dominant calf
15. Non-dominant foot

*Throughout, 'chair' can be read as 'bed'.

---

refers to an elevation in physiological activity (increased heart rate, respiration rate, resting muscle activity, etc.), cognitive arousal refers to the maintenance or perseverance of an active state of thinking. For the cognitively aroused person with insomnia, pre-sleep thoughts may be pleasant, unpleasant or emotionally neutral. The important point is that such thoughts are intrusive, and difficult to stop, engaging the thinker in further and further levels of cognitive activity. Thus, cognitive arousal may be experienced as reflecting, planning, problem-solving, or worrying.

A metaphor is useful here. When it comes to sleep, the mind is a bit like a restaurant waiting to close up. The doors are not usually locked until the last customer has left, so the exact time of closing might vary from night to night. Pre-sleep cognitions are customers who dawdle over coffee, or just refuse to leave, keeping the restaurant open later and later. The longer the restaurant stays open, the greater the chance of a new (and unwelcome) customer straying in. Similarly, the more we lie awake (for whatever reason) the more opportunity there is to think and to worry.

Cognitive arousal and sleep

Evidence that poor sleepers are more cognitively aroused (e.g. Borkovec 1982) has led to the formulation of a cognitive arousal theory of chronic insomnia, according to which sleep onset is delayed when cognitive activity is high. Several studies have reported the tendency for insomniacs to complain of intrusive, uncontrollable pre-sleep thoughts which, though not in themselves wholly negative or depressive, can substantially delay sleep onset (see Borkovec 1982, Espie 1991 for reviews). The impact of cognitive intrusions on sleep onset was demonstrated by Gross & Borkovec (1982) who recorded sleep onset latency (SOL) among groups of college students who were told either that they would have to present a speech on awakening, or that they would have to present a speech *on a particular topic* on awakening. In the first group, the experiment introduced elements of a performance anxiety; in the second (speech-and-topic) group, however, this anxiety was augmented by the opportunity to think about the given topic. The SOL was twice as high in the speech-and-topic group.

Given the contribution of cognitive activity to insomnia, and the demonstrated efficacy of relaxation treatment for insomnia, the possibility exists that relaxation methods may work, not so much through their ability to relax the body, but rather through their ability to focus the mind, reduce mental tension, and prevent intrusive thoughts. Such a possibility was explicitly recognised by Bootzin & Nicassio (1978) who refer to some relaxation procedures as *cognitive relaxation strategies*. It is also possible that such cognitive effects may be enhanced by the direct physiological impact of muscle-tone reduction, which is known to alleviate sleep-inhibiting factors like postural tension and pain. Experimental studies (reviewed by King 1980, and Borkovec 1982) clearly indicate that, while the total relaxation 'package' is associated with the best outcomes among those presenting with insomnia, individual components within the 'package' (e.g. attention focusing alone; tension–release components alone), can significantly improve sleep onset latency. The pleasant, monotonous rhythmic pattern of the relaxation itself also appears to be soporific.

Precisely how each component of relaxation training influences sleep onset remains a subject for detailed research. Nevertheless, where sleeplessness is accompanied by tension recognisable to the patient (hospital inpatients, for example, may, for a variety of reasons, experience stress), then relaxation procedures offer a practical and effective therapeutic tool. Two relaxation procedures will be considered here: progressive relaxation (or PMR); and autogenic training.

PROGRESSIVE RELAXATION TRAINING
Offering progressive relaxation training

In recent years, relaxation procedures, particularly progressive muscle relaxation, have been popularised as a means for responding to general stress, and 'relaxation packages' (containing tapes, information, and/or written instructions) are now widely available. It is important to emphasise, however, that in the context of a systematic approach to insomnia management, quality control rests with the clinician (in this case, the supervising nurse), and that progressive relaxation is better *taught* than *prescribed* (as a tape or book). If a commercially available package is used, then some degree of training, supervision and monitoring remains appropriate.

At this stage in management, it is also assumed that sleep hygiene and stimulus control interventions have already been considered, and appropriate steps taken. Relaxation procedures are well suited to patients who are confined to bed, experiencing pain, or who are, for whatever reason, anxious. Prior to offering progressive relaxation, however, it would be worthwhile first to enquire whether patients have their own preferred relaxation method for coping with stress (for example yoga or meditation). Next, given the emphasis placed on muscle tensing, it would also be appropriate to consider the suitability of patients for progressive relaxation. Where local injury, vulnerability or pain (e.g. fractures, infusion sites, postoperative wounds) make such muscle tensing unwise, these specific muscular areas may be omitted. However, where a generalised sensitivity exists (e.g. in patients with arthritis), alternative relaxation procedures should be considered. It is for this reason that, in addition to progressive relaxation, the method of autogenic training (Bootzin & Nicassio 1978) is also presented in this chapter.

The progressive relaxation training session

For the patient, the aim of relaxation training is to: (a) achieve a deep state of relaxation in a relatively short period; and (b) control excess tension, and the effects of excess tension (Bernstein & Given

1984). The training procedures achieve these aims by amplifying the somatic experience of muscle relaxation. Brief guidelines for trainers are provided in Box 8.2, with the relaxation procedure described in more detail below.

Box 8.2 Progressive relaxation training: guidelines for trainers

1. Decide on the appropriateness of progressive relaxation training for the particular patient; will procedures need to be modified to avoid certain areas or limbs?
2. Select an appropriate location and position (on a bed or comfortable chair). The location should be quiet enough to prevent distraction or interruption, and comfortable enough to support the head, limbs and trunk as they relax.
3. Explain the theory and practice of progressive relaxation training to the patient.
4. Focus the patient's attention on the muscle group to be relaxed.
5. Use a cue word (e.g. 'now') to initiate tension; maintaining the tension for 5–7 seconds.
6. Use a cue word (e.g. 'relax') to initiate relaxation, encouraging the structures supported by those muscles to become limp and heavy. Focus the patient's attention on the relaxing muscles.
7. Allow approximately 45 seconds before moving attention to the next muscle group.
8. Relax each muscle group in the order shown in Box 8.1.
9. Relaxation should be practised at least twice each day, preferably once in the morning before the day's routine commences, again at night-time when settling down to sleep.
10. The learned relaxation procedures should also be used to assist sleep onset during periods of intervening wakefulness.
11. Once instructed, the patient may practise using taped relaxation instructions both in the morning and at night.
12. Monitor and encourage the patient. Reinforce the message that the aim of treatment is to be more relaxed whether awake or asleep.
13. After 2–3 weeks, the patient should be able to relax on some occasions without using the tape, and may want to dispense with the tape altogether.
14. Relaxation forms only one part of a systematic approach to managing insomnia; maintain other relevant components (e.g. sleep hygiene, stimulus control).

Having decided on the patient's suitability, select an appropriate location in which to conduct the training sessions. A quiet room with a reclining chair or bed is ideal, though a cushioned, high-backed chair will suffice. It is important that the chair comfortably supports the head, limbs and trunk as they relax. If the patient is in bed, remove any bedding which might restrict movement, and help her to adopt the most comfortable semi-reclining position.

Next, explain the theory and practice of progressive relaxation training to the patient. For example: 'The relaxation method I am about to describe involves tensing and relaxing different muscle groups throughout your body. The aim is to produce a state of relaxation which occurs when the tension in the muscles is released. It is particularly important that you concentrate on the feelings which accompany tensing and relaxing. I will begin with the muscles in your hands, and end with the muscles in your feet. The whole procedure will take about 25 minutes. Before we start, I'll demonstrate each of the muscle groups in turn, and give you an opportunity to tense and relax each one. Don't tighten any of the muscles until I give you the signal: I will say NOW when I want you to tighten the muscle, and RELAX when I want you to completely relax the muscle.' (The cue words NOW and RELAX are written in upper case for emphasis; when spoken they can be emphasised softly, with the word 'relax' repeated.)

The trainer can now demonstrate, on his or her own body, each muscle group in turn, showing the patient how the group is to be tensed (see Box 8.1), asking the patient to copy, and emphasising the cue words 'now' and 'relax'. The key message is the importance of focusing attention on the muscle groups being tensed and relaxed. Once the method has been demonstrated, begin the session proper by asking the patient to close her eyes. Try to use a standard way of describing the tension/relaxation phase for each muscle. Adopt a tone of voice conducive to relaxation; speak softly, and rhythmically. For example: 'I'm going to ask you to tense the muscles in your (specify) by (as described in Box 8.1). NOW, tighten the muscle … keep it really tight … feel all the tension in that muscle … and …' (after 5–7 seconds) '… RELAX. Let go of the tension … feel the relaxation in the muscle … feel the tension flowing out of the muscle, and feel the relaxation flowing in …' (for limbs, add 'as your (limb) gets heavier … and heavier') '… making your (area or limb) more and more relaxed … concentrate on that relaxed feeling. Compare how it feels now to how it felt when it was tense.' Allow the muscle group to relax for approximately 45 seconds before moving attention to the next group. Relax each muscle group in the order shown in Box 8.1.

When the last muscle group has been relaxed for sufficient time, inform the patient that the session is now coming to a close. To avoid doing this abruptly, tell the patient that you will count backwards from four, counting softly and rhythmically until zero, then ask the patient to open her eyes and remind her of how relaxed she feels. It may be helpful to ask her to move her arms and legs before standing up, to return her to a fully awake state. The latter stages of progressive relaxation can be enhanced using imagery. For example, you may ask the patient at the beginning of the session to recall, and remember the image of a safe and peaceful place she may know, or have known in the past (perhaps a favourite holiday location, a special room, or a place in her garden). This image may then be cued by the trainer at the end of the session to maintain the feelings of relaxation and well-being. The session can then be terminated visually, asking the patient to take four 'steps' out of the image, again counting aloud.

It is possible that patients will sometimes fall asleep during a session. If this happens, wake them gently, and emphasise the connection between the relaxed state, and their sleep onset. From a sleep hygiene point of view, it would be unwise to leave patients sleeping for a significant period during the day.

It is important that the relaxation technique is practised at least daily, and always used after settling down to go to sleep at night. The technique should also be used by the patient to deal with periods of wakefulness after sleep onset. With practise, patients become more and more efficient at relaxing, with the benefits taking less and less time to achieve. One of the reasons for this is, again, conditioning, with the relaxation *procedure* becoming a cue for relaxation itself. With the acquisition of competence, sessions may be shortened by tensing limb muscle groups in pairs (hands, arms, thighs, etc. together). Initially, practise sessions will be greatly helped by the use of audio-taped instructions similar to those offered by the trainer. A written handout describing the technique and the procedure will also help. As with all other interventions, sleep diaries should be maintained throughout the treatment and follow-up periods.

AUTOGENIC TRAINING

As already mentioned, progressive muscle relaxation, with an emphasis on somatic tensing, may not be appropriate for all patients, particularly those with arthritis, or perhaps the frail. While progressive muscle relaxation is targeted at the body, auto-genic training is essentially a mental exercise during which the subject is encouraged to repeat, in a monotonous fashion, self-suggestions of physical heaviness in a particular limb, alternating with suggestions of physical warmth in that limb (Schultz & Luthe 1959). Several authors (e.g. Espie 1991) have commented on similarities between autogenic training and hypnosis; both may use the device of imagining heaviness and warmth in limbs, and both may be considered procedures for inducing deep relaxation. Indeed, the term 'autogenic' was first used by Johannes Schultz (see Schultz & Luthe 1959) to describe the trance-like states (the 'autogenic state') which resulted from forms of self-hypnosis practised by patients at the Berlin Neurological Institute in the 1930s (where Schultz worked). Established as an effective relaxation procedure, progressive muscle relaxation and autogenic training were found by Nicassio & Bootzin (1974) to be equally effective in reducing sleep onset latency and improving subjective sleep quality in a group of 30 insomniacs aged from 22–71 years. Again, it is likely that these treatments effects are mediated in large part by reductions in cognitive arousal. Nevertheless, autogenic training procedures provide a useful alternative to progressive (muscle) relaxation where the tension–relaxation cycle may be uncomfortable.

Offering autogenic training

As described by Schultz & Luthe (1959), and subsequently by Lichstein (1988), autogenic training operates best when the following four conditions are met.

1. The training session takes place in a state of comfort and reduced external stimulation (light, noise, etc.).
2. The trainee develops a state of 'passive concentration', where the individual is detached, relaxed and unconcerned about the outcome of the training procedures.
3. The trainee engages in the repetition of phrases emphasising:

   a. heaviness in the arms and legs
   b. warmth in the arms and legs
   c. calm and regular heartbeat
   d. calm breathing
   e. warmth in the solar plexus, and
   f. coolness in the forehead.
4. The trainee concentrates on the relevant limbs/parts of the body as the phrases are repeated.

In the version of autogenic training used by Nicassio & Bootzin (1974), attention to the arms and legs alone (excluding c–f above) was associated with significant benefits, while substantially reducing the length of the session. It is this version of autogenic training which will be presented here. More detailed versions of the technique can be found in Lichstein (1988) or Payne (1995).

It is an important principle of autogenic training that the individual patient or trainee is in control. For this reason, autogenic training instructions are written in the first person (see Lichstein 1988), and initially read to the trainee who repeats them (usually under his or her breath). Lichstein (1988) has suggested that the heaviness/warmth instructions are augmented with the phrases 'I feel at peace' and 'I am relaxed', and this suggestion is included in the instructions presented below.

The autogenic training session

Observing the first two 'rules' above, the session should take place in a quiet room with dimmed lighting. A bed or reclining chair is ideal (with the trainee lying back), but a comfortable supportive chair will suffice. As with progressive relaxation, the trainer adopts a gentle, soft, rhythmic tone of voice. Begin the session by asking the trainee to close her eyes and recall, and remember the image of a safe and peaceful place she may know, or have known in the past (perhaps a favourite holiday location, a special room, or a place in the garden). Ask the trainee to imagine that she is now lying there. Then, introduce the session as follows:

I am now going to ask you to focus your attention on different parts of your body in turn. First, I want to emphasise how important it is that you adopt a passive and casual attitude towards this procedure. Let the sensations of heaviness and warmth arise on their own. Don't try to force them by making an effort. Before we begin the exercises spend a little time relaxing … (allow 1–2 minutes for the trainee to settle down). Now we shall begin.

The trainer then directs the trainee's attention to individual limbs, and limbs on different sides of the body in the order shown in Table 8.1. (e.g. 'Let's begin with your right arm'; 'now let's move on to your left arm', etc.) On each occasion, the following phrases are recited by the trainer, and repeated (sub-vocally or mentally) by the trainee.

Trainer:	I feel at peace.
Trainee:	I feel at peace.
Trainer:	My right arm is heavy.
Trainee:	My right arm is heavy.
Trainer:	My right arm is heavy.
Trainee:	My right arm is heavy.
Trainer:	I feel at peace.
Trainee	I feel at peace.
Trainer:	My right arm is heavy.
Trainee:	My right arm is heavy.
Trainer:	My right arm is heavy.
Trainee:	My right arm is heavy.

Allow approximately 30 seconds for each exercise; then encourage the trainee to focus on that limb/part of the body for a further 30–45 seconds. Then move on to the next limb/part of the body using the phrases shown in Table 8.1.

Following the final sequence, you may terminate the session as follows:

Now, slowly allow yourself to become aware of the room; think about where you are. Open your eyes. Look around the room. Tell yourself you are going to feel refreshed and alert. Make a few weak fists with your hands; bend your elbows a couple of times. Now bend your knees. Stretch. When you're ready, slowly sit up.

Table 8.1   Sequence of autogenic training exercises[a]

Exercise	Limb/body part	Phrase
1	Dominant arm	My (right) arm is heavy
2	Non-dominant arm	My (left) arm is heavy
3	Both arms	Both my arms are heavy
4	Dominant leg	My (right) leg is heavy
5	Non-dominant leg	My (left) leg is heavy
6	Both legs	Both my legs are heavy
7	Limbs on dominant side of body	My (right) side is heavy
8	Limbs on non-dominant side of body	My (left) side is heavy
9	Arms and legs	My arms and legs are heavy
10–18	Repeat substituting 'warm' for 'heavy'	

When the trainee is familiar with the procedure, combine 'heavy' and 'warm'

[a]The sequence is based on the modified procedure used by Nicassio & Bootzin 1974.

Nicassio & Bootzin (1974) found that a 20- to 30-minute training period per day, followed by another when the patient was settling down to sleep at night, were sufficient to improve sleep onset latency both in the short term (i.e. 2, 3 and 4 weeks after the start of treatment), and at 6-month follow-up. Again, audio-tapes of the training sessions will assist practice at home, as also will written handouts describing the procedure. As with progressive relaxation training, sleep diaries should be maintained throughout the treatment and follow-up periods.

SUMMARY

In combination with appropriate sleep hygiene and stimulus control procedures, relaxation exercises provide a valuable strategy for reducing sleep latencies, and improving sleep quality. While these benefits have been demonstrated in controlled trials, the theoretical underpinnings of these effects remain unclear, but probably reflect an impact on both physical and cognitive arousal.

REFERENCES

Adam K, Tomeny M, Oswald I 1986 Physiological and psychological differences between good and poor sleepers. Journal of Psychiatric Research 20(4): 301–316

Bernstein D A, Borkovec T D 1973 Progressive relaxation training: a manual for the helping professions. Research Press, Champaign Ill

Bernstein D A, Given B A 1984 Progressive relaxation: abbreviated methods. In: Woolfolk R L, Lehrer P M (eds) Principles and practice of stress management. Guilford Press, New York

Bootzin R R, Nicassio P M 1978 Behavioral treatments for insomnia. In: Hersen M, Eisler R, Miller P M (eds) Progress in behavior modification. Academic Press, New York, vol 6

Borkovec T D 1982 Insomnia. Journal of Consulting and Clinical Psychology 50: 880–895

Espie C A 1991 The psychological treatment of insomnia. Wiley, Chichester

Gross R J, Borkovec T D (1982) Effects of cognitive intrusion manipulation on the sleep onset latency of good sleepers. Behavior Therapy 13: 112–116

Jacobson E 1929 Progressive relaxation. University of Chicago Press, Chicago Ill

King N J 1980 The therapeutic utility of abbreviated progressive relaxation: a critical review with implications for clinical practice. In Hersen M, Eisler R M, Miller P M (eds). Progress in behavior modification (Vol 6). Academic Press, New York

Lacks P 1987 Behavioral treatment for persistent insomnia. Pergamon, New York

Lichstein K 1988 Clinical relaxation strategies. John Wiley, New York

Monroe L J 1967 Psychological and physiological differences between good and poor sleepers. Journal of Abnormal Psychology 72: 255–264

Nicassio P, Bootzin R 1974 A comparison of progressive relaxation and autogenic training as treatments for insomnia. Journal of Abnormal Psychology 83: 253–260

Payne R A 1995 Relaxation techniques: a practical handbook for the health care professional. Churchill Livingstone, Edinburgh

Schultz J H, Luthe W 1959 Autogenic training. Grune and Stratton, New York

9

Thoughts and sleep: cognitive therapy for insomnia

Learning outcomes

The contribution of pre-sleep thoughts to the onset or maintenance of insomnia has received increasing attention in recent years. It is now widely accepted that some 'maladaptive' styles of thinking can encourage levels of cognitive arousal (discussed in the previous chapter) incompatible with sleep onset. Cognitive therapy, usefully deployed in other areas of psychological health, offers a range of therapeutic strategies for influencing maladaptive thoughts and improving sleep quality. This chapter outlines the rationale of cognitive therapy, as applied to insomnia, and presents an overview of effective treatments. Unlike Chapters 4–8 which described how to conduct assessments and treatments, the present chapter aims mainly to inform. On completing this chapter you should be able to:

- describe an 'automatic' thought
- define two types of cognitive error
- describe two cognitive therapy approaches to the treatment of insomnia.

INTRODUCTION

Cognitive therapy is based on a simple, but influential model of human behaviour (cognitive theory) which suggests that how people think about a particular situation determines both how they subsequently feel and how they subsequently behave. Consider, for example, a young man who has just invited a female work colleague out to dinner, and she declines. He may think 'she doesn't like me', and then conclude '... it's probably because I'm unlikeable'. Or he may think 'well, it was worth a try', and conclude '... we probably wouldn't have had much in common, anyway'. In the first response, both confidence and self-esteem are diminished, with obvious implications for future attempts at socialising. In the second, the psychological setback of refusal will probably be overcome. In cognitive theory, the typical pattern of thinking that people adopt in response to such events (i.e. their typical way of seeing the world) is called a schema.

Schemas help us to interpret or 'organise' our experiences and create our own subjective reality. Sometimes, however, the thoughts which contribute to our schemas can be systematically distorted, producing a view of the world which is unhelpful or *negative*, and which in turn results in feelings which are maladaptive or inappropriate. If, for example, a situation is erroneously interpreted as threatening, maladaptive feelings of anxiety will result. Alternatively, if situations are repeatedly interpreted as hopeless, feelings of depression may follow. (In this way, the schemas of a depressed person operate like a pair of dark glasses through which the world is viewed.) Cognitive theory (as proposed by Beck et al 1979) suggests that both the emotional and physical symptoms of pathological anxiety and depression have their origins in these cognitive distortions.

According to cognitive theory, the thoughts which contribute to habitual negative schema (and hence, negative emotions) eventually become *automatic*, coming into play before an alternative (and, perhaps, more positive) thought has an opportunity to develop. While regarded by the individual as both accurate and plausible, automatic thoughts are in fact characterised by distortions of thinking described by Beck et al (1979) as 'cognitive errors' or 'cognitive distortions'. Typical cognitive distortions are presented in Table 9.1. Cognitive therapy aims to reduce the impact of dysfunctional or negative schemas by helping individuals to modify the influence of automatic thoughts. This may be achieved directly, by helping individuals to identify and challenge their automatic thoughts, or it may be achieved indirectly by distracting or otherwise preventing (blocking) the development of such thoughts. Examples of cognitive therapies are summarised in Table 9.2. While these techniques have been widely used in the treatment of anxiety and depression, experience has shown that they are also well suited to the management of some sleep problems.

Table 9.1 Cognitive errors (distortions) which support negative schemas

Name	Definition
Overgeneralisation	Forming general conclusions from evidence which is too narrow, and too specific (for example, concluding from a single argument 'everybody hates me')
Arbitrary inference	Forming specific conclusions without adequate evidence, or in spite of *contrary* evidence (for example supposing yourself to be a terrible time-keeper on the basis of a single missed appointment)
Selective abstraction	Focusing on a single detail taken, out of context, from a given situation
Magnification and minimisation	Under- or overrating the significance of specific events and experiences
Personalisation	Tendency to relate external events to oneself when there is no evidence of a direct connection
Dichotomous thinking	The tendency to place events into all-or-none categories (for example, in relationships, seeing oneself as either totally in control, or totally powerless, but without anything in between)

Table 9.2 Cognitive therapy approaches to the management of insomnia

Type of therapy	Description
Didactic	Reducing pre-sleep anxieties and arousal by improving the patient's knowledge of sleep and the consequences of sleep loss
Pre-emptive	Avoiding pre-sleep cognitive arousal by rescheduling pre-sleep problem solving and/or rehearsing constructive responses to possible pre-sleep anxieties
Thought-blocking and distraction	Preventing the development of pre-sleep cognitive arousal, using techniques which inhibit anxiety-laden thinking
Cognitive restructuring	Confronting the automatic thoughts which promote pre-sleep cognitive arousal, challenging these thoughts and replacing them with positive, realistic alternatives
Paradoxical intention	Reducing the anxieties associated with frustrated sleep onset by 'prescribing the symptom' (i.e. recommending that the patient stays awake as long as possible.

Cognitive therapy and insomnia

As mentioned in Chapter 8, pre-sleep thoughts which promote cognitive arousal may be positive, negative or emotionally neutral. What makes them counterproductive to sleep onset is that they are intrusive, difficult to stop, and engage the thinker in further and further levels of cognitive activity. It is also possible that, whatever their original content, such thoughts may ultimately acquire emotional significance (i.e. they can become worrisome or upsetting), leading to what has been termed *emotional arousal* (Espie 1991). Sometimes the pre-sleep emotions of people experiencing chronic insomnia are related to the consequences of their own poor sleep. Thus, people may worry about how lack of sleep will affect their performance the next day; or they might become disheartened by their repeated inability to 'do something as simple as fall asleep'.

Whether neutral, or typically associated with anxiety or depression, cognitive therapy provides a range of strategies which can prevent or interrupt maladaptive and perseverative thoughts and thereby lower cognitive arousal and promote sleep onset. However, unlike the relaxation therapies which have been extensively researched since the early 1970s, the application of formal cognitive therapy procedures to insomnia is less well established, and the evidence of efficacy is continuing to develop. Nevertheless, cognitive therapies have been found effective in the treatment of older insomniacs (Morin & Azrin 1988), chronic insomniacs (Espie et al 1989), and clinically heterogeneous insomniac groups (Morin et al 1994). While effective both alone (Espie et al 1989) and in combination with relaxation therapies (Morin & Azrin 1988), the evidence does suggest that the benefits from some cognitive approaches may be less robust, and more variable than the benefits from others (see Lacks & Morin 1992).

The emphasis here on *formal* cognitive therapy is important. Other treatment approaches (e.g. relaxation, health education), though not explicitly practised as cognitive therapies, may nevertheless exert an influence on sleep through cognitive arousal. As suggested in Chapter 8, relaxation strategies, in addition to reducing physical tension, almost certainly affect the individual's ability to entertain intrusive cognitions. Viewed in this way, then, progressive muscle relaxation can be regarded as a form of thought-blocking cognitive therapy. Similarly, health education may help to reduce or remove unrealistic (and anxiety-provoking) expectations of sleep which, as the content of an intrusive cognition, may have prolonged sleep onset latencies.

COGNITIVE THERAPY APPROACHES TO INSOMNIA

In the non-pharmacological treatment options presented in Figure 4.1 (p. 63), and described in Table 4.1 (p. 64), cognitive therapy is identified as a high-skills intervention requiring both specialised training, and appropriate supervision. Such training is, however, well within the ambit of a post-registration nurse. In this section, therefore, cognitive approaches to sleep problems are described only in brief. It is hoped that the information will be of value both to those unfamiliar with the techniques of cognitive therapy, and those who may be accustomed to the technique, but who may be unaccustomed to its use in the management of insomnia. Five different 'cognitive' treatment approaches will be considered here. With the possible exception of didactic approaches (see below), the aim of cognitive therapy is to enskill the patient, encouraging competence in the techniques through initial learning sessions with the clinician, and daily homework sessions alone.

Didactic approaches

As already emphasised, anxiety can be an important cause of excessive cognitive arousal and consequent delayed sleep onset. Where anxieties about sleep and sleeplessness are directly related to an individual's unrealistic assumptions about, and expectations of sleep, appropriate sleep education (as described in Ch. 6) can play an important role in reducing such cognitive arousal. The value of simple sleep education measures, therefore, in reducing sleep anxieties should not be overlooked. Often, however, worries about the likely consequences of sleep loss, or anxieties about not getting 'enough' sleep, reflect a more fundamental tendency to 'misattribute' all daytime ills to poor night-time sleep. In the latter case, additional cognitive approaches may be necessary.

Pre-emptive approaches

Since the aim of cognitive therapy is to reduce cognitive arousal during the *pre-sleep period*, and thus encourage sleep onset, one logical way to approach the issue would be to reschedule the individual's usual pre-sleep thinking (or pre-sleep worrying) for earlier in the day. For example, individuals may be encouraged to set aside a period each day just to consider issues that worry them (a so-called 'worry-buffer'), while agreeing not to entertain these thoughts at night. Espie & Lindsay (1987) suggest an approach termed 'worry control' where, in addition to spending time each day identifying current anxieties, the patient is also asked to identify constructive responses to each of these anxiety-provoking problems. Then, if thoughts about these problems arise during sleepless periods in bed, the patient is encouraged to intercept the worry with a reminder that things are 'in hand'.

Thought-blocking and distraction

These approaches aim to deal with intrusive thoughts by removing them from the mental agenda, either by blocking them altogether, or by distraction (in effect, by changing the subject). Blocking techniques can range from counting sheep (perhaps the oldest, but least recognised as such, cognitive therapy for poor sleep) to the repetition of pre-arranged mantras which can accompany meditation (Woolfolk et al 1976). An alternative to the mantra (with its emphasis on rhythmical repetition) has been termed 'articulatory suppression' (Levey et al 1991), and involves repeating a particular word at *irregular* intervals (for example, the word 'the'), thus occupying the patient with a cognitive task (try it).

While blocking procedures operate to prevent all coherent (including intrusive) thinking, distraction offers the mind an alternative, more adaptive train of thought. Some of the relaxation methods already considered in Chapter 8 contain an implicit cognitive distraction element (for example, repeating to oneself the progressive muscle relaxation procedure instructions). Imagery training (also mentioned in Ch. 8) where individuals recall tranquil, safe and pleasant scenes, can also be used to distract the thinker from intrusive and negative thoughts and improve sleep onset (see Morin & Azrin 1988).

Cognitive restructuring

As already mentioned, some patients appear to have a problem controlling their pre-sleep thoughts and find it difficult to get into the right frame of mind for going to sleep. For these people, relaxation may work because, by providing a focus of attention, it prevents or blocks the typically automatic and maladapative thoughts which can delay sleep onset. An alternative way of dealing with these same thoughts has been termed 'cognitive restructuring'. The aim here is not to avoid or block thoughts but to meet them head-on, learn to recognise them for what they are (such thoughts will often be characterised by one or more of the cognitive errors shown in Table 9.1), challenge them, and ultimately replace them with more reassuring and rational alternatives. This three-stage approach (capturing thoughts; challenging thoughts; replacing thoughts) requires careful introduction by the therapist, and considerable practice by the patient, and is outlined in the instructions reproduced below.

Offering cognitive restructuring for insomnia

The following introductory steps to cognitive restructuring for insomnia have been suggested by Morgan & Gledhill (1991) and provide an overview of this approach to treatment. These instructions can be offered on written handouts, but only as an adjunct to more in-depth sessions conducted by an experienced practitioner. These steps are reproduced here only to illustrate the process of treatment.

Whether preoccupied with the past, ruminating on the present or anticipating the future, our thoughts affect how we feel and what we do. For example, consider Mr A, an elderly widower who is used to sharing a holiday each year with his son's family. This year they haven't invited him. What might he think?

1. Maybe they are fed up with me always being around. I must be boring company for them. Have I done something to offend them? They have stopped caring about me. Or
2. They have been considerate to take me with them in the past. I can understand that they need time together as a family. Maybe it's good for me to know I can manage without them.

If he believes [the first] train of thoughts he would probably feel sad, angry or puzzled. He may even feel like avoiding his family or become irritable in their company, and whenever such thoughts revisit him. If he believes [the second] train of thoughts he is less likely to feel upset. He may even feel pleased for not putting himself first.

Consider a further example: Mr A has now been asked by a relatively new acquaintance to go on holiday together. What might he think?

1. I'm not sure what I'm committing myself to. We might have different tastes. We might not get on. What if we were to fall out? Or,
2. I'm reluctant to go on holiday alone. Perhaps this is a good opportunity for me. We might get on well. I am still free to make up my own mind about the things I would like to do.

If he believes [the first] train of thoughts he would probably feel anxious and keep dwelling on the things that could go wrong, even worrying that it could end up disastrously. These thoughts might well disrupt his sleep. If he believes [the second] train of thoughts he is more likely to feel comforted, even pleased. These thoughts are unlikely to disturb his sleep.

Remember.   What you say to yourself affects how you feel and what you do. The things you say to yourself at night-time can make you emotionally aroused and keep you awake. Once started, these thoughts are very difficult to stop, and you may find yourself becoming more anxious, sad or angry. So by stopping the spiral of these unpleasant and unhelpful thoughts at times when you are in bed, you can encourage a more restful sleep.

Identifying automatic thoughts.   Having explained some of the basic rationale of cognitive therapy, the practitioner can then introduce the importance of identifying automatic thoughts.

The aim of this treatment is to help you to deal with the kinds of thoughts that may be keeping you awake at night. First, you must learn to identify your disruptive thoughts so that you can challenge them. Often these thoughts, which are called *automatic* thoughts, will have one or more of the following features:

- They are automatic and habitual; they just seem to pop up without any effort on your part.
- They are irrational or distorted: they do not always fit the facts.
- They are exaggerated: they tend to overestimate danger or difficulty.
- They are unhelpful: they keep you anxious, depressed or angry.
- They are plausible: it may not occur to you to question them.
- They are involuntary: they can be very difficult to 'switch off'.
- They are defeatist: they presume you cannot possibly cope.

At first you may not find it easy to catch your automatic thoughts, but with practice it will become more natural. Once you have learned to spot an automatic thought, you can then learn to provide yourself with an alternative which is more realistic and positive.

To practice:

1. Set aside 25 minutes each evening to make a record of your thoughts. Do this at least two hours before going to bed.
2. Write down everything you can remember thinking in bed last night. Try to record these as accurately as possible. Write them down word for word if you can. If your thoughts take the form of pictures rather than words, write down what you saw in your 'mind's eye'.
3. Now examine each thought you have written down. Is it realistic? Can you think of something to replace it with? What would you say to a friend with this thought? Write your conclusions down in the next column, and decide how much you believe in the thought now.

Beware of excuses which keep you from focusing on your thoughts or writing your diary. It is quite natural to avoid recalling unpleasant thoughts or experiences. However, doing so is one of the best ways of controlling an overactive mind, and encouraging restful sleep.

Restructuring thoughts.   Further sessions can then focus upon actually restructuring the patient's automatic thoughts.

As we discussed earlier, what you say to yourself, your impressions and thoughts, can affect how you feel and what you do. Certain automatic thoughts can help to keep you awake. If this happens you can improve your sleep first by identifying these automatic thoughts, and then by changing them. Once you have identified an automatic thought, consider two types of question.

1. What evidence is there that this thought is true?
   a. Are you confusing thought with fact? Just because you believe something to be true doesn't mean it *is* true.
   b. Are you jumping to conclusions? If you are, then you are basing your conclusions on poor evidence.
   c. Examine the evidence for your particular thought. What evidence do you have to back it up? Do you know anything that might contradict your thought? Do you think this particular thought would be accepted by other people?
2. What alternatives are there to this particular thought? Suggest some and consider:
   a. What is the evidence to support an alternative thought?
   b. How do you think another person would see things?
   c. What might you say to another person if they told you about this thought?

After examining the thought and producing an alternative, try to think of a statement which sums up the alternative view. Recall this statement if the original thought arises when you are trying to get to sleep.

To practice:

1. Set aside 25 minutes each evening and repeat the exercises described above in which you identify your automatic thoughts.
2. This time, examine each thought and ask yourself the questions: what is the evidence? and what are the alternatives?
3. Having worked through the above steps you should now produce a short positive statement which reassures you. Make sure it is one you can believe. If you can't find one, go back and examine the original thought again; look at the evidence and produce an alternative.

When you go to bed at night you may find you have thoughts which you have already worked on during the day. If so, remember the positive reassuring statement you produced. Even if it is a new thought you will probably be able to use these reassuring statements. Try repeating them to yourself while thinking of a pleasant relaxing scene. You will probably find that the thought does not come into your mind again and sleep will shortly follow. If your reassuring statement doesn't reassure you, then you will have to work through the thought again as you did in the exercise during the day.

Sleep-specific thoughts and insomnia

Cognitive restructuring, as described so far, addresses all kinds of negative, automatic and intrusive thoughts which might arise during the pre-sleep period, and thus frustrate sleep onset. Morin (1993), however, has emphasised that the 'automatic' pre-sleep thoughts of those experiencing insomnia are often sleep specific, typically reflecting (in addition to the cognitive errors defined in Table 9.1) unrealistic expectations (of sleep onset times or optimal sleep duration) and misattributions (a false belief that much of what goes wrong in an individual's day is directly caused by poor sleep). Identifying and addressing these sleep-specific errors of thinking should, therefore, be a priority of the restructuring process as well as a target for initial education.

Paradoxical intention

In addition to being intrusive and negative, sleep-specific thoughts can also generate anxieties which become self-fulfilling. Thus, anxieties about not being able to sleep will lead to higher levels of cognitive arousal which, of course, will delay sleep onset, and so on. Where such thinking has come to typify the individual's sleep problem, an alternative cognitive approach to treatment is the use of a technique called 'paradoxical intention'. The basic rationale of this approach is elegantly simple. Anxieties resulting from unsuccessful attempts to fall asleep can be reduced (and sleep onset encouraged) by instructing the patient to *stay awake*. Originally proposed as an effective treatment for sleep onset insomnia by Ascher & Efran (1978), more recent studies have continued to demonstrate its value in some, but not all patients (Espie & Lindsay 1985). A detailed critique of the clinical efficacy of paradox, together with precise instructions on its use, can be found in Espie (1991).

Cognitive therapies: general

As with other approaches to sleep management, the impact of cognitive therapies should be monitored throughout the treatment period, with appropriate encouragement given at follow-up appointments. Cognitive therapy requires a considerable commitment from the patient in terms of home-based practice (so called 'homework'). It is in the interests both of the patient and the clinician, therefore, that a trusting, professional alliance is established early in treatment which maximises adherence, and optimises treatment outcome.

REFERENCES

Ascher L M, Efran J S 1978 Use of paradoxical intention in a behavioral program for sleep onset insomnia. Journal of Consulting and Clinical Psychology 46: 547–550
Beck A T, Rush A J, Shaw B F, Emery G 1979 Cognitive therapy of depression. Guilford Press, New York
Espie C A 1991 The psychological treatment of insomnia. Wiley, Chichester
Espie C A, Lindsay W R 1985 Paradoxical intention in the treatment of chronic insomnia: six case studies illustrating variability in therapeutic response. Behaviour Research and Therapy 23: 703–709
Espie C A, Lindsay W R 1987 Cognitive strategies for the management of severe sleep-maintenance insomnia: a preliminary investigation. Behavioural Psychotherapy 15: 388–395
Espie C A, Lindsay W R, Brooks D N, Hood E M, Turvey T A 1989 controlled comparative investigation of psychological treatments for chronic sleep-onset insomnia. Behaviour Research and Therapy 27: 79–88
Lacks P, Morin C M 1992 Recent advances in the assessment and treatment of insomnia. Journal of Consulting and Clinical Psychology 60: 586–594

Levey A B, Aldaz J A, Watts F N, Coyle K 1991 Articulatory suppression and the treatment of insomnia. Behaviour Research and Therapy 29: 85–89

Morgan K, Gledhill K 1991 Managing sleep and insomnia in the older person. Winslow Press, Bicester

Morin C M 1993 Insomnia – psychological assessment and management. Guilford Press, New York

Morin C M, Azrin N H 1988 Behavioral and cognitive treatments of geriatric insomnia. Journal of Consulting and Clinical Psychology 56: 748–753

Morin C M, Culbert J P, Schwartz S M 1994 Nonpharmacological interventions for insomnia: a meta analysis of treatment efficacy. American Journal of Psychiatry 151: 1172–1180

Woolfolk R L, Carr-Kaffashan L, McNulty T F, Lehrer P M 1976 Meditation training as a treatment for insomnia. Behaviour Therapy 7: 495–503

Hypnotic drugs in the treatment of insomnia

Learning outcomes

As indicated in Figure 4.2 (p. 66), hypnotic drugs have an important role in the treatment of some insomnias. This chapter examines the nature, effects, and side-effects of hypnotic drugs, and considers the optimal use of these drugs in the management of insomnia. On completing this chapter you should be able to:

- name three factors determining the duration of activity of hypnotic drugs
- explain what is meant by a 'double-blind' clinical trial
- describe two effects that hypnotic drugs have on sleep
- provide two reasons for advising intermittent hypnotic drug consumption.

INTRODUCTION

The word 'hypnotic' stems from the Greek *hypnos* meaning sleep. In Greek mythology, a minor deity of the same name – Hypnos – flitted between Hades and the living world exerting his soporific influence on mortals and immortals alike. In clinical pharmacology, a drug is described as a hypnotic if it promotes sleep. (Used in this context, the term 'hypnotic' should not be confused with the trance-like state popularised in the late 18th century by Friedrich Anton Mesmer. The hypnotic trance, so called because of its supposed similarity to sleep-walking, is in fact misnamed since hypnosis is not a state of sleep.) In addition to promoting sleep, most hypnotic drugs reduce anxiety. Hypnotics and tranquillisers are, therefore, the same in virtually everything but name.

History and hypnotics

The medicinal value of naturally occurring substances which can relieve pain and sleeplessness has long been recognised in human societies, and the poppy *Papaver somniferum* has, for at least the past 2000 years, provided a rich source of pain-killing and sleep-inducing preparations. From this single plant come opium, heroin, morphine, laudanum, and other 'opiates', each of which can induce sleep if taken in sufficient quantities. Unfortunately, these drugs also interfere with other essential functions like breathing or the reflex mechanism which makes us cough. As an alternative to such naturally occurring (but rather dangerous) substances, research chemists and pharmacologists in the 19th and 20th centuries turned their attention to the manufacture of compounds that were safe to use and specific in their action, affecting sleep and little else. One of the first 'true' hypnotic drugs, chloral hydrate, was synthesised in 1832 and introduced towards the end of the 19th century. Chloral derivatives continue to be used today. In 1903 the first barbiturate drugs were introduced, which, throughout the first half of the 20th century, became the most widely used of all hypnotics. Barbiturates, however, were addictive, widely abused, and often fatal in overdose. Because of these disadvantages (and the introduction of the safer benzodiazepines), barbiturates fell from favour and are now rarely used in the treatment of insomnia.

Most of the hypnotics and tranquillisers currently prescribed belong to the benzodiazepine group. Introduced in the early 1960s, benzodiazepines soon replaced the more toxic and more habit-forming barbiturates as the drugs of choice for treating both anxiety and sleeplessness. The first of these new anxiolytics (or 'tranquillisers'), chlordiazepoxide, was developed by Roche Laboratories in Europe and was first introduced into the USA under the trade name 'Librium' in 1960. Soon to follow were diazepam (Valium) in 1963 and nitrazepam (Mogadon), the archetypal benzodiazepine hypnotic, in 1965. While benzodiazepines have dominated the drug management of insomnia for over 3 decades, concern about their widespread use, and the problems of 'normal dose dependency' (see Lader 1994) have resulted in a progressive decline in prescriptions for benzodiazepines. Nevertheless, most benzodiazepines currently prescribed in the UK are prescribed as hypnotics rather than tranquillisers (see Fig. 2.8, p. 36). In the 1980s, two new, non-benzodiazepine hypnotics were introduced, the cyclopyrrolone zopiclone and the imidazopyridine zolpidem. Described as a new generation of hypnotics (e.g. Musch & Maillard 1990), both drugs show some advantages over the benzodiazepines, and are consequently increasing in popularity. The therapeutic effects and side-effects of contemporary hypnotic drugs are summarised in Box 10.1 and discussed below.

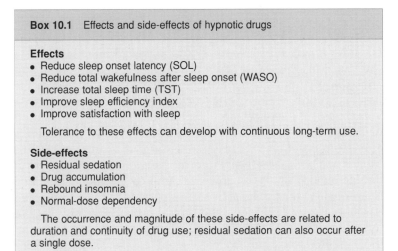

Box 10.1   Effects and side-effects of hypnotic drugs

Effects
- Reduce sleep onset latency (SOL)
- Reduce total wakefulness after sleep onset (WASO)
- Increase total sleep time (TST)
- Improve sleep efficiency index
- Improve satisfaction with sleep

  Tolerance to these effects can develop with continuous long-term use.

Side-effects
- Residual sedation
- Drug accumulation
- Rebound insomnia
- Normal-dose dependency

  The occurrence and magnitude of these side-effects are related to duration and continuity of drug use; residual sedation can also occur after a single dose.

EFFECTS OF HYPNOTIC DRUGS ON SLEEP

Unlike those drugs developed in the late 19th or early 20th century, benzodiazepines, and the more recent zopiclone and zolpidem, were introduced at a time when sleep, and the impact of drugs upon sleep, could be accurately and precisely measured. As a result, there now exists a detailed sleep laboratory profile for most of the hypnotic products currently prescribed. The procedure most usually employed to assess the effects of a new hypnotic drug is the clinical trial, during which the sleep of volunteers is recorded polysomnographically before, during and after a course of sleeping tablets. To avoid the introduction of bias encouraged by expectations, such trials employ what is called a 'double-blind' procedure, which means that in addition to the real or 'active' hypnotics, the volunteer also takes inactive dummy tablets which look like, and should taste and smell like, the active drug. Active and dummy hypnotics are then administered in a sequence known only to a third person, leaving both the volunteer and the researcher 'blind' to the nature of each tablet. On completion of the trial, the researcher learns when active and dummy drugs were taken, and codes the EEG sleep recordings and all other experimental data accordingly. By convention, the dummy drug is referred to as a 'placebo', the Latin for 'I will please'.

Effective hypnotic drugs reduce sleep onset latency, decrease the amount of wakefulness intervening during sleep, and consequently increase total sleep time. Figure 10.1, for example, shows the results from a double-blind trial of a typical benzodiazepine taken for a period of 3 weeks by middle-aged poor sleepers. In this study, placebos were taken before (the 'baseline' period) and after (the withdrawal period) the active drug. Relative to the baseline period, which can be considered as the norm for these volunteers, the measurements obtained during the 3-week period of drug taking show a marked reduction in total wakefulness after sleep onset (WASO). Hypnotic drugs also affect subjective satisfaction with sleep. Daily records maintained by volunteers in double-blind drug trials show clear improvements in subjective sleep quality during the active drug periods relative to placebo baseline. Figure 10.2 shows the typical influence of an effective hypnotic on daily visual analogue ratings of sleep quality. Again, the baseline week can be considered as the norm for these volunteers. Satisfaction with sleep shows a dramatic improvement after the first dose of active hypnotic, and is maintained at an elevated level until the drug is withdrawn.

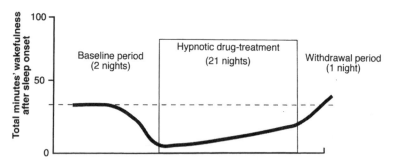

Figure 10.1   Impact of a typical intermediate half-life benzodiazepine hypnotic on total wakefulness after sleep onset (WASO). Relative to the baseline period (the norm for these middle-aged poor sleepers), WASO shows a marked reduction during the active drug period, followed by a moderate 'rebound' on the first withdrawal night. (Based on Adam et al 1984.)

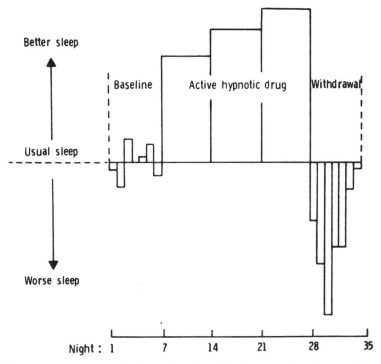

Figure 10.2   Impact of a typical intermediate half-life benzodiazepine hypnotic on daily visual-analogue ratings of sleep quality. Relative to the baseline period (the norm for these middle-aged poor sleepers) subjective sleep quality is increased throughout the active drug period (averaged weekly ratings), but decreased immediately following withdrawal. Note also that these subjective reports do not reflect tolerance. (Source: Morgan et al 1984.)

Duration of action

Unlike most other drugs used in clinical practice, hypnotics are required to act only for a limited period within the 24-hour cycle. Pharmacological activity which continues beyond this period can be considered as an undesirable effect (or a side-effect) of the drug. As we shall see in the next section, sedation which persists into the next day is a serious complication of hypnotic drug use. It follows, therefore, that some understanding of the duration of action of hypnotics is essential when caring for patients taking night-time sedation.

The duration of activity of a given hypnotic is determined by three factors: absorption; distribution; and elimination. The rate at which the drug is absorbed from the gut into the circulation determines the onset of drug action, with the more rapidly absorbed drugs acting sooner. Once absorbed, the drug is then distributed via the bloodstream to organs, tissues and cells within the body. This process of distribution necessarily results in a fall in the plasma concentration of drug. Plasma levels then continue to fall as the drug is progressively metabolised and excreted. These three phases of drug action are shown in Figure 10.3. While rates of absorption and distribution vary considerably from one hypnotic to another, duration of hypnotic drug action is primarily influenced by the rate of elimination. The most widely used measure of the elimination phase is the elimination half-life or elimination $t_{1/2}$ (i.e. the time taken for the plasma concentration of a drug to halve once the distribution phase is complete). Hypnotic products differ widely in their elimination $t_{1/2}$, and may be categorised as having long, intermediate, or short half-lives (see Table 10.1).

Figure 10.4 shows hypothetical plasma concentrations for two hypnotics with similar absorption and distribution profiles, but differing elimination half-lives. While both products would have a similar impact on sleep onset, the longer-acting drug would continue to influence sleep much later into the night, and possibly influence behaviour the following day. In addition, while some hypnotics are inherently longer acting than others, the speed with which the drug is eliminated from the system frequently depends on the age of that system. In general, since older bodies are less

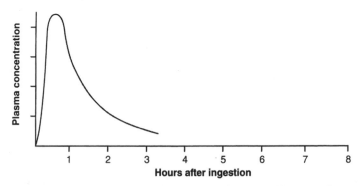

Figure 10.3 Hypothetical plasma concentrations for a typical hypnotic. Peak concentrations are reached when the drug is maximally absorbed; concentrations then decline rapidly as the drug is distributed to the various body 'compartments'; a slower decline then follows as the drug is metabolised and cleared.

Table 10.1 Half-lives of typical benzodiazepine, and non-benzodiazepine hypnotic drugs

Drug	Half-life (hours) of drug or active metabolites (h)
Long half-life	
Diazepam	24–100
Flurazepam	50–100
Nitrazepam	20–40
Intermediate half-life	
Lorazepam	12–20
Temazepam	10–17
Oxazepam	12
Lormetazepam	13–14
Loprazolam	15
Short half-life	
Triazolam	3
Zopiclone	5
Zolpidem	2
Midazolam	2–7

Sources: Bianchetti et al 1988, Gaillot et al 1983, Hugget et al 1981, Humpel et al 1979, 1980, Jochemsen et al 1983a, b, Lader 1983

efficient than younger bodies at eliminating drugs, elimination half-lives tend to be prolonged in elderly people. Greater care is therefore required when sleep problems in later life are managed with hypnotics (see Morgan 1990).

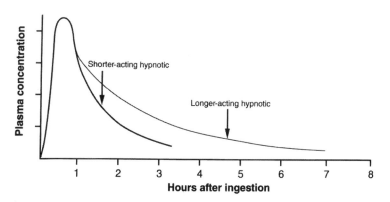

Figure 10.4 Hypothetical plasma concentrations for two hypnotics with similar absorption and distribution profiles. The longer-acting drug would continue to influence sleep much later into the night, and might produce residual sedation the following morning.

Finally, it should be noted that for some hypnotics, the elimination half-life of the main constituent may not give an accurate indication of that drug's likely duration of action. During the elimination phase, drugs are broken down by the body into more easily excreted 'metabolites'. Some of these metabolites may themselves be active hypnotics which persist longer than the parent compound. Both diazepam and flurazepam, for example, release the active metabolite N-desmethyldiazepam, a sedative drug with a half-life of approximately 100 hours.

Tolerance

While hypnotics improve sleep quality in the short term, this effect can diminish if the drug is taken regularly over long periods. In many cases, such regular use produces 'tolerance' whereby the body becomes accustomed to the drug, larger doses of which are then required in order to achieve the original effect. In the UK, these effects were recognised in benzodiazepines as early as 1980, when the Committee on the Review of Medicines (a body set up under the Medicines Act of 1968 to assess the safety, quality, and efficacy of drugs marketed in the UK) concluded that 'Most hypnotics tend to lose their sleep-promoting properties within three to 14 days [of continuous use]' (Committee on the Review of Medicines 1980). Some degree of tolerance is clearly shown in Figure 10.1. Throughout the 3 weeks of drug ingestion, WASO gradually moves towards its baseline (pre-drug) level. Nevertheless, it is well recognised in clinical practice that for some patients, long-term benzodiazepine use may not be associated with obvious signs of tolerance (Lader 1994, National Medical Advisory Committee 1994). One explanation for this discrepancy is the difference between subjective and objective measures of tolerance phenomena. Note, for example, that in Figure 10.2, volunteers appeared to become more, not less satisfied with their sleep as the trial progressed (but were nevertheless clearly dissatisfied with their sleep during withdrawal). Furthermore, it is also important to acknowledge that few long-term benzodiazepine users increase their drug dosage to maintain the same pharmacological effect. For this reason, the terms 'normal dose' or 'therapeutic dose' dependency have been used to describe typical long-term benzodiazepine addiction (Lader 1983).

BEHAVIOURAL SIDE-EFFECTS OF HYPNOTICS

In addition to being effective as sleep-inducers, benzodiazepines, and other recently introduced hypnotics, have proved extremely safe, even when taken in massive overdose. These drugs can, however, be associated with profound, and sometimes quite dangerous *behavioural* side-effects, the most important of which will be considered here.

Residual effects

Ideally, hypnotics should be active only during the hours of sleep. Unfortunately, this apparently simple requirement is not always met and the sedative action of some hypnotics can persist after waking, influencing and disrupting daytime activities. Various terms have been used to describe these effects, including 'hangover effects', and 'residual effects'. The term 'residual effects', will be used here since 'hangover' traditionally refers to the consequences of drug *withdrawal* (as with alcohol) rather than drug persistence.

Residual effects can be additive. It was noted above that drugs with a long half-life tend to remain active in the body longer than drugs with a shorter half-life. Some hypnotics persist for so long that traces of the drug are still present at the following bedtime. If such a hypnotic is taken on two consecutive nights, peak concentrations of the second dose will be added to residual concentrations of the first, leading to even higher residual concentrations the next day. In this way, residual amounts of the drug can accumulate so that daytime behaviour, perhaps unaffected after a single dose, can be affected after several consecutive doses.

First reported for benzodiazepine hypnotics by Bond & Lader (1972), residual effects arising from sleeping drug use have long been recognised. In an essay 'On the Use of Hypnotic Drugs in the Treatment of Insomnia' published in the *Journal of Mental Science* in 1905, for example, Dr W Maule Smith identified one of the main characteristics of drug-induced sleep as being 'The inability of the parts acted upon by the drug to free themselves from the enforced restraint due to the lingering effect of the hypnotic'. Dr Smith went on to note that 'The degree of this effect varies with the constitution of the drug and the dose prescribed'. As also mentioned above, ageing bodies become less efficient at clearing drugs from the system. In elderly users, therefore, hypnotics tend to persist longer, and daytime behaviour disruptions due to the 'lingering' effects of these drugs become more likely. In addition, residual drug effects in the elderly may be superimposed upon existing age-dependent reductions in mental and physical efficiency. Consequently, among elderly users, residual effects are not only more likely, but can also be more profound.

Residual effects at any age can range from gross daytime sedation to more subtle disruptions of behavioural efficiency (e.g. impaired coordination, judgement, and memory) detectable, in laboratory tests, in users who do not feel sedated, and who are not overtly drowsy (see Morgan 1994, Woods et al 1987, 1992). In epidemiological studies hypnotic drug consumption has been associated with reduced work performance, absenteeism (Jacquinet-Salord et al 1993), and road traffic accidents (Jacquinet-Salord et al 1993, Leger 1994, Ray et al 1992) in the general population. Among elderly people, hypnotics (Ray et al 1987, Wysowski et al 1996) have also been specifically implicated as causes of falls and fractured neck of femur. Such risks are amplified in patients concomitantly receiving daytime medication with sedative effects (e.g. sedative antidepressants, daytime anxiolytics, antihistamines, some analgesics, etc.).

Rebound effects

Drugs that alter mood and behaviour (i.e. psychotropic drugs) can often affect the body not only when they are present, but also when they are withdrawn. Alcohol provides a good example of this; taken in large amounts, its presence may be associated with feelings of well-being, while its withdrawal may be accompanied by the malaise of hangover. In the case of hypnotics, drug withdrawal can be associated with characteristic 'rebound' effects, i.e. 'temporary changes from baseline that are the opposite of those initially produced by the drug' (Woods et al 1987). Three types of rebound will be considered here: rebound insomnia; REM rebound; and rebound anxiety.

Rebound insomnia

As already mentioned, regular hypnotic usage can be associated with tolerance, whereby the body becomes accustomed to the drug, larger doses of which are then needed in order to achieve the original effect. In practice, larger doses of hypnotic benzodi-azepines are not usually taken and the sleep-inducing properties of the same repeated dose can diminish over time. In addition, the regular consumption of benzodiazepine hypnotics is also associated with the development of dependence, as evidenced by the occurrence of withdrawal effects (however mild) when the drug is withdrawn. Conceptually, the presence of the drug is making the body 'push' much harder in the direction of greater sleepless-ness in order to maintain its usual level of functioning. If a benzodiazepine to which tolerance has developed is abruptly withdrawn, then all resistance to these adaptive changes is removed, and what was compensation in the presence of the drug becomes overcompensation in its absence. Following regular usage, therefore, withdrawal of some benzodiazepine drugs is followed by a disturbance of sleep referred to as 'rebound insomnia'.

The onset and severity of rebound effects will depend upon the speed at which the drug is eliminated from the body. Thus, the withdrawal of shorter-acting drugs produces an earlier rebound than the withdrawal of long-acting drugs. Indeed, some long-acting drugs like flurazepam take so long to leave the system that rebound effects are not observed. In such cases, the notion of 'abrupt' with-drawal is, perhaps, inappropriate (i.e. since some drugs may persist for days, ingestion that is abruptly discontinued does not result in plasma or tissue levels which abruptly decline). Rebound insomnia is clearly shown in Figure 10.1 for the first withdrawal night follow-ing 3 weeks of continuous drug ingestion. In most cases, the body rapidly adjusts, with levels of intervening wakefulness returning to the pre-drug (baseline) levels after 3–7 nights. Figure 10.2, for example, clearly shows that while the withdrawal of the active drug is associated with a sharp decline in subjective sleep quality, this effect is short-lived. It is important, therefore, that rebound insomnia is not interpreted as a recrudescence of pre-drug symp-toms. Certainly, long-term hypnotic drug users should be advised not to discontinue their drugs abruptly (see Box 10.2).

REM rebound

Hypnotics also affect the overall structure of sleep, reducing total amounts of both REM and stage 4 sleep. On withdrawal of the drug, REM sleep can also rebound, sometimes to well above pre-drug levels. As dreams are most likely to occur during the REM

Box 10.2 Prescribing hypnotic drugs: general considerations (Lader 1992, National Medical Advisory Committee 1994)

- Before prescribing, the *aetiology* of the problem should be clarified, and the likely *duration* of the problem should be estimated.
- Depressed patients should usually be treated with an antidepressant. In those who are agitated as part of the depression, a sedative antidepressant is preferable to the concomitant use of a hypnotic.
- Phenothiazines should be avoided as treatments for insomnia.
- All (benzodiazepine) hypnotics carry the risk of dependence; patients should be advised of these risks.
- Select the hypnotic with care. Shorter-acting drugs are more likely to cause withdrawal effects; longer-acting drugs are more likely to cause residual/accumulation effects.
- Prescribe the lowest effective therapeutic dose.
- Treatment should initially be limited to 1–4 weeks.
- Hypnotic drugs should be reviewed on a regular basis, and discontinued as soon as possible.

---

stage, this rebound can be associated with vivid dreaming and sometimes nightmares. Once again, the rebound effect subsides as the body readjusts to the absence of the drug.

Rebound anxiety

It has already been mentioned that in addition to promoting and maintaining sleep, hypnotics can also reduce anxiety. In fact, hypnotic and tranquillising drugs are virtually identical. Where poor sleep is associated with stress and anxiety, a longer hypnotic drug may be prescribed especially to exploit its residual anxiolytic effects during the day. With repeated use, tolerance to these tranquillising effects also develops such that, on withdrawal, anxiety can 'rebound' above pre-drug levels.

Rebound effects: conclusion

Although they are transient, rebound effects have serious implications for both successful withdrawal and the well-being of long-term hypnotic drug users. For those who wish to discontinue their hypnotics but who are unaware of, or unable to cope with, the immediate consequences, a short period of rebound insomnia accompanied perhaps by increased daytime anxiety may be enough to convince them that they need their sleeping tablets after all. In this way, many people may continue to take their hypnotics not to promote sleep per se, but rather to avoid the unpleasant consequences of withdrawal. These problems can be overcome with reassurance and advice, a gradual 'tapering off' of drug usage and, where appropriate, non-pharmacological treatment for the underlying insomnia.

DRUG MANAGEMENT OF INSOMNIA

There is now widespread agreement that 'hypnotic medication should not be the mainstay of management for most of the causes of disturbed sleep' (National Institutes of Health 1991), and that 'further effort is needed to review the use of benzodiazepines and replace them, as necessary, with behavioural, cognitive, and psychotherapeutic methods' (DoH 1992). Nevertheless, hypnotics do have an important role to play in the management of short-term and, perhaps, intermittent insomnias where the daytime consequences of such disturbance are 'severe, disabling, or subjecting the individual to extreme distress' (Committee on Safety of Medicines 1988). Where drug management is appropriate, shorter half-life drugs (at the lowest possible dose) are clearly preferable, with intermittent use encouraged, and a limited 'course' of drugs prescribed.

Useful guidelines on the integrated (psychological and pharmacological) management of insomnia have been published in the UK by Lader (1992) and the National Medical Advisory Committee (1994). Some of the principal recommendations from these reports are summarised in Box 10.2, and in the algorithm shown in Figure 4.2 (p. 66). Both documents stress the value of hypnotic drug use in the context of a broader treatment plan. Since most of the disadvantages associated with hypnotic drugs are related to duration of usage, a critical role for the acute unit or community nurse is to monitor drug use and respond when short-term use (say, 2–3 weeks) looks set to graduate to long-term use. Ultimately, such monitoring and caution are doubly in the patient's favour: first by avoiding unnecessary side-effects; and second by preserving the impact of an important therapeutic for perhaps subsequent use. In both the hospital and community setting, therefore, drug therapy for insomnia introduces some special nursing issues which are summarised in Box 10.3. It is important, however, that the nurse recognises that hypnotics represent just one of a range of effective treatment options which may be offered in parallel with, or instead of, drug therapy.

Box 10.3 Hypnotic drug use: nursing considerations

Drug administration
Most hypnotics are prescribed p.r.n. (i.e. to be taken when necessary).
The need for night sedation should always be discussed with the patient,
and the disadvantages of chronic use made clear. Where possible,
encourage intermittent use. This will help to preserve the pharmacological
impact of these extremely useful drugs.

Knowledge
Different hypnotic drugs can have very different durations of action.
The nurse administering a hypnotic should be aware of that drug's
elimination half-life, and the likelihood of residual sedation and possible
accumulation following from its use.

Observation
The elimination half-life of many hypnotics is increased in disease, and in
older age groups. Some shorter-acting drugs may, therefore, cause
sedation, impaired performance, or instability the following day. The use
of hypnotics among the ambulant ill and frail should be accompanied by
increased supervision during the day.

Review and discharge
Hypnotics commenced in hospitals are often continued in the community
following discharge. To avoid unnecessary use, discuss the need for
such medication with the patient; make hypnotics a special target for
pre-discharge drug reviews. Where hypnotics have been consumed
regularly (i.e. nightly) over long periods, abrupt withdrawal should be
avoided, and gradual reduction advised.

Primary caregiving and hypnotic drug prescribing

Several factors have already been mentioned which make
hypnotic drugs very special. For example, they are required to
work only for a limited period within the 24-hour cycle, with
continued activity representing a serious side-effect. In addition,
they are drugs of dependence which may be associated with
disturbing rebound effects; yet, as p.r.n. drugs, the patient is
invested with full responsibility for initiating withdrawal.
(Remember that, if prescribed as *tranquillisers*, benzodiazepines
are consumed in divided daily doses, and are discontinued only
by the prescribing physician.) From a nursing point of view, two
other factors make these drugs quite distinct. First, hypnotics are
frequently prescribed for a condition (insomnia) which is neither
directly observed, nor investigated by the prescribing physician.
Instead, prescribers often rely either on the (daytime) reports of

patients or, not infrequently, on the daytime or night-time reports of primary caregivers. Where nurses are the primary caregivers, their observations can directly influence prescribing.

Second, hypnotics can easily be prescribed for *situations* rather than *individuals*. Consider, for example, a twin-bedded room or bay in a hospital or nursing home where one patient is restless and perhaps noisy at night, while the other, disturbed by the noise, is complaining. Assuming that, on clinical grounds, hypnotics are not contraindicated, could not this situation be improved by prescribing a hypnotic (albeit short term and at the appropriate dosage) for either patient? This hypothetical (but, we believe, not too far-fetched) example serves to illustrate the sometimes narrow line separating individual need, and institutional need in the prescription of some hypnotics. This issue is of considerable clinical and social importance in relation to older patients in non-hospital residential establishments, where high levels of hypnotic drug prescribing can be a cause for concern (see Alessi et al 1995, Buck 1988, Middelkoop et al 1994, Seppala et al 1993, Snowdon et al 1995). Acknowledging both of these factors helps to identify a special role for the nurse who, as primary caregiver, can, and should, influence both the likelihood and the appropriateness of hypnotic drug prescribing. Explicit recognition of this role is an important step towards the improved sleep management of inpatients and nursing home residents.

REFERENCES

Adam K, Oswald I, Shapiro C 1984 Effects of loprazolam and triazolam on sleep and overnight urinary cortisol. Psychopharmacology 82: 389–394
Alessi C A, Schnelle J F, Traub S, Ouslander J G 1995 Psychotropic medications in incontinent nursing home residents: association with sleep and bed mobility. Journal of the American Geriatrics Society 43: 789–792
Bianchetti G, Dubruc C, Thiercelin J P, Bercoff E et al 1988 Clinical pharmacokinetics of zolpidem in various physiological and pathological conditions. In: Sauvanet J P et al (eds) Imidazopyridines in sleep disorders. Raven Press, New York, pp 155–163
Bond A J, Lader M H 1972 Residual effects of hypnotics. Psychopharmacologia 25: 223–235
Buck J A 1988 Psychotropic drug practice in nursing homes. Journal of the American Geriatrics Society 36: 409–418
Committee on Safety of Medicines 1988 Benzodiazepine dependence and withdrawal. Current Problems 21: 1–2
Committee on the Review of Medicines 1980 Systematic review of the benzodiazepines. British Medical Journal 280: 910–912

Department of Health 1992 Health of the nation: a strategy for health in England. HMSO, London

Gaillot J, Heusse D, Houghton G W et al 1983 Pharmacokinetics and metabolism of zopiclone. Pharmacology 27: 76–91

Huggett A, Flanagan R J, Cooke P, Crome P, Corless D 1981 Chlormethiazole and temazepam. British Medical Journal 282: 475

Humpel M, Illi V, Milius W, Wendt H, Kurowski M 1979 The pharmacokinetics and biotransformation of a new benzodiazepine (lormetazepam) in humans. 1. Absorption, distribution, elimination and metabolism of lormetazepam-5-14 C. European Journal of Drug Metabolism and Pharmacokinetics 4: 237–243

Humpel M, Neiuweboer B, Milius W, Hanke H, Wendt H 1980 Kinetics and biotransformation of lormetazepam. ii. Radio-immunologic determinations in plasma and urine of young and elderly subjects: first-pass effect. Clinical Pharmacology and Therapeutics 28: 673–679

Jacquinet-Salord M C, Lang T, Fouriaud C, Nicoulet I, Bingham A 1993 Sleeping tablet consumption, self reported quality of sleep, and working conditions. Journal of Epidemiology and Community Health 47: 64–68

Jochemsen P A, van Rijn T G M, Hazelzet C J, van Boxtel C J, Breimer D D 1983a Comparative pharmacokinetics of midazolam and loprazolam in healthy subjects after oral administration. In: Jochemsen R (ed) Clinical pharmacokinetics of benzodiazepine hypnotics. J H Pasmans, 's-Gravenhage, pp 176–83

Jochemsen R, van Boxtel C J, Hermans J, Breimer D D 1983b Pharmacokinetics of 5 benzodiazepine hypnotics in the same panel of healthy subjects. In: Jochemsen R (ed) Clinical pharmacokinetics of benzodiazepine hypnotics. J H Pasmans, 's-Gravenhage, pp 81–94

Lader M H 1983 Dependence on benzodiazepines. Journal of Clinical Psychiatry 44: 121–127

Lader M (ed) 1992 The medical management of insomnia in general practice. Royal Society of Medicine Round Table Series 28. Royal Society of Medicine, London

Lader M 1994 Benzodiazepines – a risk–benefit profile. CNS Drugs 5: 377–387

Leger D 1994 The cost of sleep-related accidents: a report for the National Commission on Sleep Disorders Research. Sleep 17: 84–93.

Middelkoop H A M, Kerkhof G A, Smilde-Van Den Doel D A, Ligthart G J, Kamphuisen H A C 1994 Sleep and ageing: the effects of institutionalisation on subjective and objective characteristics of sleep. Age and Ageing 23: 411–417

Morgan K 1990 Hypnotics in the elderly: what cause for concern? Drugs 40: 688–696

Morgan K 1994 Hypnotic drugs, psychomotor performance and ageing. Journal of Sleep Research 3: 1–15

Morgan K, Adam K, Oswald I 1984 Effects of loprazolam and triazolam on psychological functions. Psychopharmacology 82: 389–394

Musch B, Maillard F 1990 Zopiclone, the third generation hypnotic: a clinical overview. International Clinical Pharmacology 5(suppl 2): 147–158

National Institutes of Health 1991 Consensus development conference statement: the treatment of sleep disorders of older people. Sleep 14: 169–177

National Medical Advisory Committee 1994 The management of anxiety and insomnia. HMSO, Edinburgh

Ray W A et al 1987 Psychotropic drug use and the risk of hip fracture. New England Journal of Medicine 316: 363–369

Ray W A, Gurwitz J, Decker M D, Kennedy D L 1992 Medications and the safety of the older driver: is there a basis for concern? Human Factors 34: 33–47

Seppala M, Rajala T, Sourander L 1993 Subjective evaluation of sleep and the use of hypnotics in nursing-homes. Aging – Clinical and Experimental Research 5: 199–205

Smith W M 1905 On the use of hypnotic drugs in the treatment of insomnia. Journal of Mental Science 51: 561–575

Snowdon J, Vaughan R, Miller R, Burgess E E, Tremlett P 1995 Psychotropic-drug use in Sydney nursing-homes. Medical Journal of Australia 163: 70–72

Woods J H, Katz J L, Winger G 1987 Abuse liability of benzodiazepines. Pharmacological Reviews 39: 251–419

Woods J H, Katz J L, Winger G 1992 Benzodiazepines: use, abuse, and consequences. Pharmacological Reviews 44: 151–347

Wysowski D K, Baum C, Ferguson W J, Lundin F, Ng M J, Hammerstrom T 1996 Sedative-hypnotic drugs and the risk of hip fracture. Journal of Clinical Epidemiology 49: 111–113

Sleep management within special groups

Learning outcomes

This chapter is concerned with the sleep of special groups of people. At different times of life, and under particular circumstances, normal sleep may change. Discrete events such as pregnancy may produce temporary changes, while ongoing processes such as ageing may be associated with gradual and permanent changes. On completing this chapter you should be able to:

- describe two changes in sleep associated with pregnancy and the early stages of motherhood
- name three risk factors associated with sudden infant death syndrome (SIDS)
- name three causes of sleep disturbance particular to older adults
- describe three strategies to minimise the effects of working night-shifts.

INTRODUCTION

There are several special groups of people whose sleep may be of concern to nurses. For most of these, sleep may be unsatisfactory due to normal physiological changes or voluntary changes in behaviour. Internal events such as the ageing process and hormonal changes can disturb the quality and or quantity of sleep. Behavioural changes such as travel and undertaking shiftwork are likely to produce difficulties in adjusting sleep to a different time schedule. These groups are discussed here.

WOMEN AND SLEEP

Pregnancy

Pregnancy is a time when sleep is temporarily disrupted for most women and these disturbances are most profound during the last 3–4 weeks. Changes in sleep usually persist into the first few weeks following delivery. While pregnant women have problems in both initiating and maintaining sleep, postpartum women still tend to have problems in maintaining sleep, but not in falling asleep (Lee & DeJoseph 1992).

Three main factors are of concern: sleep duration and quality; insomnia; and daytime alertness. In the first trimester, sleep duration and quality and insomnia are worst and the most commonly cited reasons for this are heartburn, nausea and vomiting. Later, in the third trimester, increased insomnia and decreased daytime alertness are worst. The most frequent complaints are restless sleep, urinary frequency, fetal movement, low back pain, leg cramps and frightening dreams (Hertz et al 1992, Suzuki et al 1994). During the week before labour, women report poorest sleep effectiveness and highest sleep disturbance (Evans et al 1995).

Back pain in late pregnancy can be caused by prolonged lying in the supine position. This position frequently leads to obstruction of the vena cava, producing hypoxaemia leading to backache. This might then lead to compromised metabolic supply to neural structures, resulting in pain. That pain, if sufficiently severe, may well disturb sleep (Fast & Hertz 1992).

Finally, the quality of sleep varies according to whether it is a first or subsequent pregnancy. Primigravidae tend to experience more disturbed sleep with an approximately 12% fall in sleep efficiency (third trimester compared with postpartum). Multigravidae only show a 4% fall in efficiency (Waters & Lee 1996).

Pregnancy, then, is associated with disrupted sleep, although the causes vary according to the stage of pregnancy. Midwives are in the best position to inform mothers-to-be about possible changes in sleep, and their causes. They can advise on expectation of sleep and the use of non-pharmacological approaches to nausea reduction, such as drinks containing ginger (see Table 11.1). Similarly, they can teach non-pharmacological approaches to sleep promotion (see Ch. 6).

Table 11.1   Nursing interventions to help women with their sleep

Problem	Nursing intervention
Sleep disrupted by pregnancy	Advise mothers-to-be on what to expect, i.e. the possibility of heartburn, nausea and vomiting in the first trimester; urinary urgency, fetal movement, cramps and backache in the third trimester
	The use of drugs such as anti-emetics and hypnotics is inadvisable during pregnancy. Hot drinks incorporating ginger act as mild anti-emetics
	Backache can be reduced by careful positioning in bed with the use of extra pillows as support
Sleep disrupted by neonate	Keeping the infant in the same room as the mother, or sometimes bed sharing can minimise night-time disturbances for breastfeeding mothers
	When bottle-feeding, partners of mothers can take over feeding for short (or long) spells to allow the mother time to sleep. Even short naps during the day can help
Sleep disrupted by the menopause	Inform women of what to expect, and reassure about normal changes. If the woman wishes, refer to GP for hormone therapy if problems are severe

Motherhood

Postpartum sleep varies considerably between individuals. There has been some debate about whether staying in hospital or going home after delivery allows the greatest opportunities for sleep. In either situation, sleep is frequently disturbed by the need to empty the bladder as well as episiotomy discomfort. Other less influential factors include emotional changes such as anxiety and elation, endocrine changes, the chronic effect of prenatal sleep pattern disruption and medication use (Lentz & Killien 1991).

Although it is commonly thought that staying in hospital takes the pressure off new mothers, the hospital environment is rarely quiet and restful (see Ch. 12). A study which compared the sleep of postnatal mothers who had short or longer stays in hospital illustrated this point. Those who went home within 3 days or less were compared with those who stayed in longer than 3 days. There were few differences between the groups in terms of the hours slept, night-time awakenings, and feelings of tiredness (Carty et al 1996). This suggests that going home sooner rather than later does not necessarily mean that women will be more tired as a result. For all of these women, nevertheless, tiredness was a major factor in their experience, regardless of length of stay.

Poor sleep has been associated with postnatal depression, although it is not necessarily a causative factor. At 2–3 postpartum weeks, there is no clear relationship between tiredness and the onset of depression, but there is a clearer association between the extent of tiredness and the degree of established depression (Entwisle & Doering 1981).

The main causes of sleep disturbance among postpartum women are simply the demands of childcare. In the early stages of mother-hood there may be many disturbances for feeding during the night. The extent of the disruption can be minimised by keeping the baby close to the mother at night. Bottle-feeding mothers may be able to delegate feeding to their partners on occasion. Apparently parent–infant bed-sharing is not uncommon in the UK. It is generally thought that such arrangements are detrimental to the sleep of parents, but research does not show this to be the case. It appears to have only a slight impact on the sleep of mothers, reducing total sleep time by about 4% (Mosko et al 1997).

The menopause

The menopause is associated with changes in sleep. Hormonal changes producing hot flushes appear to be the main cause of this, but there may be other physiological changes involved (Shaver et al 1988). During and after a hot flush, body heat is lost rapidly, and then shivering frequently occurs as a way of producing the necessary heat to restore normal body temperature.

The thermoregulatory disruption which produces hot flushes has knock-on effects on the quality of sleep and may be associated with chronic sleep disturbance. Although there is an increase in the amount of stage 4 sleep, the first period of REM is shortened and episodes of wakefulness occur (Woodward & Freedman 1994). The frequencies of both hot flushes and night-time awakenings can be reduced by oestrogen therapy (Erlik et al 1981).

Nurses and midwives have a clear role in advising women on sleep changes associated with childbearing and the menopause (see Table 11.1).

CHILDREN AND SLEEP

Neonates

Sleep patterns may be detected in the brain activity of the fetus. It is not until 36 weeks' gestation, however, that this electrical activity becomes clearly defined. Premature babies, who are born before 36 weeks show higher proportions of rapid eye movement (REM) and lower proportions of non rapid eye movement (NREM) than older infants, but they also show a greater amount of indeterminate sleep. At birth, neonates have approximately equal amounts of REM and NREM sleep, and a shorter REM–NREM sleep cycle, at 50–60 minutes compared with 60–90 minutes in adults. For normal full-term babies, the average sleep time per 24 hours is 13–16 hours. As the baby gets older, the proportion of REM sleep diminishes and shifts towards the latter third of the night. Although it takes several months for circadian rhythms to become fully developed, the beginnings of 24-hour synchronicity are already present in the neonate (Sadeh et al 1996).

During the first month after birth there is a period of central nervous system reorganisation during which sleep, wakefulness and other physiological variables undergo substantial changes. Babies begin to develop circadian rhythmicity and synchronise their circadian sleep–wake cycle with 24-hour environmental cues. From 1–3 months they have a polyphasic sleep–waking pattern, initially based on 4-hourly feeding. This begins to develop into a diurnal pattern. The diurnal sleep–wake rhythm emerges by 3 months and by 6 months, the largest portion of sleep takes place during the night. This process may be deliberately encouraged by reinforcing environmental zeitgebers, such as ensuring regular changes in light levels, and routine feeding schedules and caregiving patterns.

During the subsequent 6 months, the physiological states of sleep and wakefulness are increasingly well defined. The fine structure of NREM appears, allowing the detection of stages 1–4 of sleep. However, only about 16% of babies sleep through the night at 6 months old, about the same proportion again have no regular sleeping pattern, and the same proportion again wake more than once, about two to eight times during the night. Parents may use a variety of strategies to cope with this – for example rocking or cuddling the baby, giving the baby a dummy, and feeding with milk or another drink (Sadler 1994).

There is a range of common sleep problems which are of concern to new parents. In most cases, however, reported sleep problems are symptomatic of concerned parents who have misguided expectations of their child's sleep. On the other hand, parents' distress can signal the presence of disturbed or ill parents as well as genuine sleep problems in the infants themselves. The most common causes for anxiety about babies' sleep are the risk of sudden infant death syndrome (SIDS) and difficulty getting to sleep and waking during the night.

The possibility of SIDS is a major worry for some mothers. It generally occurs after babies have been settled down to sleep and the cause is not entirely clear. There are several putative risk factors, including sleeping with bed covers over the infant's head, on a second-hand mattress, in a smoky atmosphere, and lying prone (Fleming et al 1996). Currently the latter seems to be the strongest predictor of SIDS. Interestingly, the use of a dummy appears to have a protective effect.

Post-neonatal mortality from 1980–1992 for Australia, the UK, New Zealand, the Netherlands, Norway, Sweden and the USA has been evaluated (Willinger et al 1994). Deaths due to SIDS fell by approximately 50% over this period. The main change made by targeted populations was in the sleep position of neonates – the recommendation is to place them on their side or back, not prone.

The main sleep problems actually encountered by infants and toddlers seem to be difficulty getting to sleep, and waking during the night. A large Italian study of 2889 children showed that more than one-third of children aged 2 or less had such problems (Ottaviano et al 1996). A smaller UK study showed similarly that about one-fifth of 9-month-old children had difficulties settling down to sleep and two-fifths woke regularly during the night (Galbraith et al 1993). It seems that these disturbed sleep patterns may last for months, and sometimes for more than a year (Richman et al 1975).

Up to the age of about 3 years, children may be unhappy about being put to bed, but this is rarely due to a real disorder of sleep. Similarly, up to one-third of children may wake several times during the night, but this is usually an annoying but normal part of child development, rather than being in any way pathological. There are a few babies who sleep through the night from day one, but most wake regularly, from every 20 minutes to 6-hourly over the 24-hour day. Night-time awakenings are a normal occurrence at all ages (Anders and Keener 1985, Williams et al 1974), but for the most part this only becomes a problem when there are difficulties in getting back to sleep.

Most night-time awakenings have no pathological cause, although sometimes there are obvious physical causes such as hunger, wind and the need for a nappy change. Enlarged adenoids can lead to upper airway obstruction which may produce sleep apnoeas resulting in awakenings. After a few months, most babies do not require to be fed during the night, so hunger gradually becomes less of a problem. Babies may sleep poorly if they are suffering from an infection such as chickenpox, or if they are in pain, for example, because of earache. Most parents, however, learn to recognise when their babies are genuinely distressed, by the quality of their cries.

Some infants who wake during the night just go back to sleep, while others cry. Parents who respond to crying tend to reinforce the conditions (e.g. cuddling, rocking) required for the child to fall asleep. This kind of crying can be reduced by letting the baby learn how to go to sleep unaided. This may be done by changing the behaviour of the parents so that they stop responding to cries at night, either suddenly or as a gradual process.

Colic is another cause of crying. Colic has been poorly researched despite its prevalence, but appears to be related to central nervous system development during the first few months of life. The condition is ill-defined, but colicky infants have been described as 'otherwise healthy and well-fed [who] had paroxysms of irritability, fussing or crying lasting for a total of more than 3 hours a day and occurring on more than 3 days in any 1 week ... and that the paroxysms continued to recur for more than 3 weeks' (Wessel et al 1987). Most babies stop exhibiting symptoms of colic by 4 months. Parental mismanagement of sleep due to over-concern after this period can lead to sleep problems in older infants.

Sleepless children may cause considerable stress to their parents. Sleep-deprived parents are likely to be tired and irritable, suffering a reduction in both physical and mental well-being. Consequently, children who wake frequently and do not settle back down have been shown to be at risk of physical abuse from their parent (Bax 1980, Crawford et al 1989, Jenkins 1980, Jones & Verduyn 1983).

Behavioural approaches (see Ch. 11) to the management of problem sleep in infants and babies have been particularly successful. Thus, while few babies need to learn *how* to sleep, many apparently problem infants simply need to be encouraged to sleep *alone*. The babies of parents who are taught behavioural strategies to promote healthy, self-sufficient sleep in their offspring, can show significantly better sleeping patterns (Wolfson et al 1992). Alternatively, prevention through the giving of advice may be helpful, and has been shown to be effective in reducing the incidence of sleep problems (Kerr et al 1996). Health visitors are well placed to give this sort of advice.

Older children

The length of sleep continues to lessen as children get older. Between the ages of 6 and 12, sleep is reduced by about 1½ hours (see Table 11.2). The proportion of stage 4 sleep progressively increases throughout adolescence and then decreases as sexual maturity is reached. During adolescence there is a significant fall in waking alertness, even though the total amount of night-time sleep does not always change (Carskadon & Dement 1987). In many cases, this sleepiness is due to shortened night-time sleep as a result of increasing social activities, and the likely additive chronic sleep restriction following on from this. This is more clearly seen in college students, who tend to accrue a sleep deficit during the week, and take extended sleep at weekends. However, it does not appear that pubertal sleepiness is always linked to shortened sleep.

Nocturnal enuresis (bed wetting) affects about one in six children aged 5 or less. Although it is predominantly a problem for younger

Table 11.2 Normal mean overnight sleep parameters in healthy children aged 6–11 years (adapted from Coble et al 1987, pp. 32–33)

Parameter (mean values)	6- to 7-year-olds	8- to 9-year-olds	10- to 11-year-olds
Time spent asleep	547 min	514 min	467 min
Number of REM periods	5.8	4.8	4.2
% REM sleep	20.7%	22%	19.8%
% slow wave sleep (stages 3 and 4)	24%	21.8%	21%
Number of arousals	3.2	2.7	1.6

Table 11.3 Nursing interventions for sleep problems with children

Problem	Nursing intervention
Neonates not adjusting to the 24-hour day	Provide time cues linked to desirable diurnal patterns, e.g. light during the day, dark at night; most care, bathing, etc. during daytime
Possibility of sudden infant death syndrome (SIDS)	Ensure that babies lie on their backs in their cot. Do not use second-hand mattresses or place blankets over the babies' heads
Infants and toddlers having difficulty getting to sleep and waking during the night	Advice to parents before problems occur. Behaviour modification
Nocturnal enuresis	Reassure parents that this is unproblematic in children aged approximately 5 years or less. Refer for assessment and treatment if necessary in older children

children, it can continue into the teenage years (Thomas 1997). Children usually grow out of it without any special intervention. Narcolepsy, although rare, usually appears during puberty or later. These two conditions are discussed more fully in Chapter 3. Again, nurses have an important role (Table 11.3). The kinds of sleep problems encountered among infants may be dealt with, at least in the first instance, by health visitors. Problems in older children may be less likely to come to the attention of nurses, unless the child is admitted to hospital. It may be, however, that practice nurses have a role to play here.

OLDER PEOPLE AND SLEEP

Age-related changes in sleep structure and depth

As already shown in Chapters 1 and 2, the sleep of older people, relative to that of the young, is characterised by more frequent and longer nocturnal awakenings, reductions in total sleep time, and reductions in the deeper stages of sleep. It has also been shown that auditory awakening thresholds (i.e. the minimum amount of noise required to wake a sleeping subject) are significantly reduced among older age groups (Zepelin et al 1984). In later life, therefore, sleep appears shorter, lighter, more broken, and more vulnerable to disruption. Disturbances of the sleep–wake cycle, such as those which result from transmeridian travel (Preston 1973), shift work (Monk 1992) or sleep deprivation (Webb, 1981) are also less well tolerated by older people.

However, given that in later life structural changes in sleep are experienced by the majority, while complaints of unsatisfactory sleep quality are expressed by the minority (see Chapter 2), it is reasonable to conclude that age-related change per se is not a sufficient condition for the development of insomnia. Rather, the evidence clearly points to the existence of additional factors which can help to initiate, or maintain, a severe sleep problem in later life. Since, in both secondary and community care settings, older people may have a relatively large amount of contact with nursing services, some of the more influential factors associated with late-life sleep disturbance are listed in Box 11.1, and briefly summarised below. Suggested nursing responses to these problems are listed in Table 11.4.

Box 11.1 Factors influencing sleep quality in later life

Age-related changes in sleep structure and depth

Physical health
- General symptoms (including nocturia)
- Sleep related respiratory disturbance
- Periodic leg movements (nocturnal myoclonus)

Mental health
- Dementia
- Depression

Institutionalisation
Social circumstances

Physical health

General symptoms

Acting singly, or in combination with other risks and influences, health and social status factors can have a profound impact on sleep quality, with physical ill health (Gislason and Almqvist 1987) and psychosocial status (Dew et al 1994) increasingly being recognised as influential concomitants of insomnia in old age. In a survey of health and disturbed sleep conducted among over 3000 elderly people living in rural Iowa, USA, for example, Habte-Gabr et al (1991) found that limitations of physical function, self perceptions of health, joint pain and stiffness, emphysema, and a history of stroke or heart disease were all significantly associated with poor quality, unrefreshing sleep.

Nocturia

The need to empty the bladder during the night (nocturia) becomes quite common in later life. About 60% of women and about 70% of men aged over 65 leave their beds at least once during the night to go to the toilet (Brocklehurst et al 1971). In itself, this is not a problem; most people can cope with one or two night-time excursions. Getting up for the toilet can become a problem if, on returning to bed, the individual experiences difficulty in getting back to sleep.

Periodic leg movements and Sleep related respiratory disorders

It has long been assumed that age-related changes in the structure of human sleep (as described above) reflected aspects of 'normal ageing'. However, the possibility has now arisen that some of these apparently normal changes may be related to Sleep related respiratory disorders (SRRD) or Periodic leg movements (PLM), awareness of which has grown rapidly in recent years. Both SRRD and PLM are extremely prevalent in later life (see Chapter 3), and are known to be disruptive of sleep continuity and quality. Whether, and to what extent, these conditions have 'contaminated' earlier normative studies of human sleep, or whether structural changes in sleep predispose the individual to SRRD and PLM or vice versa, remains unknown (see Bliwise, 1993).

Mental health

Dementia

Dementia presents a special area of concern in late life sleep disturbance, since many of the polygraphic sleep changes seen in normal aged individuals, and described above, are amplified in dementing illness. Relative to age-matched controls, older people with dementia take longer to get to sleep (Allen et al 1987) wake up more frequently during the night (Allen et al 1987; Prinz et al 1982), stay awake longer when disturbed (Prinz et al 1982), tend to be more active during periods of wakefulness (Allen et al 1987), and in one study, were found to be up to 20 times more likely to fall asleep during the day (Prinz et al 1982). Changes in the circadian organisation of *total* sleep have also been reported. In a detailed comparison of demented and non-demented inpatients, Allen et al (1987) found that patients with dementia not only slept more during the day, but that some (10%) actually slept more during the day than during the night (so called day-night reversal).

These changes in the architecture and circadian timing of sleep, often accompanied by episodes of night-time agitation and wandering (or 'sundowning' (Bliwise 1993) contribute substantially to the demands of caring and are among the most frequently cited reasons for the breakdown of caregiving in the community (Gilhooly 1984; Gilleard 1986; Pollak and Perlick 1991).

Whatever the organic origin, it is likely that the disruption of sleep in dementia is exacerbated by behavioural factors. The research evidence clearly indicates that regularising day-time and night-time activities, optimising daytime stimulation, minimising daytime naps, and maximising the psychological association between the bedroom and sleep all make significant contributions to the maintenance of satisfactory sleep–wake cycles in non-demented insomniacs. In dementing illness, however, the influence of these and other factors may be greatly diminished or lost. For example, a demented patient with severely disturbed night-time sleep may be left to nap ad lib during the day by an exhausted relative. As a result, the patient may be less tired and less likely to sleep during the night, which in turn can lead to sleepiness and excess napping the following day, and so on. Support for the general proposition that behavioural factors exacerbate sleep fragmentation in dementia can be found in the clinical literature. Hinchcliffe et al (1991) for example, describe the successful management of dementia-related night-time sleeplessness and wandering through stimulating daytime 'distractions' which prevented excessive napping.

Depression

At all ages, depression frequently produces an insomnia characterised by increased sleep fragmentation and early morning awakening, to the extent that symptoms of disturbed sleep are important diagnostic features of clinical depression. In laboratory studies of depressed elderly people, the degree of sleep disturbance has been correlated with the severity of the underlying depressive illness (Reynolds et al 1988). Depression must, therefore, be considered as an important cause of sleep disturbance in later life (Morgan 1996). Nevertheless, it should also be remembered that, in old age, the prevalence of insomnia greatly exceeds the prevalence of depression, making it unlikely that overall levels of the former are primarily due to the latter. While insomnia affects between a quarter and a third of all elderly people living at home (see Chapter 2), estimates suggest a community prevalence of depression in this age group of approximately 9–10% (Morgan 1996). Where insomnia is associated with an underlying depression, improved sleep quality generally accompanies successful treatment (Walsh et al 1994).

Institutionalisation

As evidenced by levels of hypnotic drug use (Morgan 1990) or reported sleep problems (Middelkoop et al 1994), institutionalisation represents a major risk factor for disturbed sleep in later life. Outwith factors associated with the need for admission (pain, anxiety, bereavement, etc.), several mechanisms can be identified which mediate this risk. The first night in unfamiliar surroundings often results in sleep which is shorter, lighter, and more broken, a phenomenon described as the 'first night effect' (Agnew et al 1966; Scharf et al 1975). All other things being equal, sleep returns to its normal pattern after a few nights. It is possible, however, that during this vulnerable time, other factors may influence successful adaptation. Excessive daytime napping (often through boredom) has been identified as an important source of circadian disruption in nursing homes (Ancoli-Israel et al 1989) while noise levels represent a major cause of night-time disturbance in both hospitals and nursing homes (see Chapter 3).

Social circumstances

Finally, an individual's personal circumstances can often have a marked effect on sleep quality. Retirement, financial limitations, bereavement and the social response to illness can all affect sleep in later life. It is, therefore, important to acknowledge the possibility that disruptions of sleep in older patients do not always result from illness or irreversible biological change, but may be the result of adverse personal or environmental circumstances. Loneliness and social isolation, for example, can produce feelings of vulnerability and fear which antagonise sleep onset. Financial hardship, on the other hand, may result in inadequately heated houses, or the use of older beds and bedding, which may contribute to, and exacerbate, age-related sleep fragmentation.

Table 11.4 Nursing interventions for sleep problems in older people

Problem	Intervention
Unrealistic expectations of sleep	Explain normal changes in sleep associated with ageing
Pain and physical discomfort	Ensure that pain is controlled as well as possible, either by analgesic medication or through other strategies such as relaxation, limb supports and careful positioning
Changes in bladder function	Encourage regular habits and ensure that diuretics are taken at the correct time
Sleep disordered breathing	Refer to GP if problematic
Anxiety and depression	Ascertain cause, refer to GP if appropriate
Bereavement, loneliness	Nurses may provide pointers for making other social contacts: e.g. lunch clubs, university of the third age, light voluntary work, etc
Poor sleeping environment due to financial difficulties	Advice on economic methods of keeping warm, social work referral if necessary
Institutionalisation	Keep environment quiet at night, try to allow elderly people to follow the same routines as they would follow at home

SHIFTWORKERS

Factory workers, police and nurses are the groups most often studied for the effects of shiftwork on sleep. The requirement of working nights may pose problems for some which are not encountered by others, and individual factors have a powerful influence on the ability to adapt. However, a greater understanding of the problems of working nights can help managers and workers to minimise them.

Our circadian rhythms have evolved so that our bodies are alert and active during the day and asleep during the night. Night shifts disrupt the internal and external cues which entrain us to a normal 24-hour environment. Night work is tolerated well by some, and is an endurance test for others; in retrospect, many individuals perceive their experience of working nights as being worse than they realised at the time (Spelten et al 1993).

Shiftwork and circadian rhythms

Sudden changes in the patterns of sleeping and wakefulness are not instantly compensated for by our inbuilt diurnal rhythms. It takes weeks for these rhythms to resynchronise. Different physio-logical rhythms (such as body temperature, cortisol secretion and the sleep–wake cycle) adjust at different rates, and the desynchro-nisation of these different rhythms experienced during this process can produce negative effects on health in many people. Some individuals are unable to make complete adjustments, even over longer periods of time.

Night-shift workers often have problems sleeping which result from this desynchronisation. About 60–70% of shiftworkers report sleep disruption (Rutenfranz et al 1985). There is a strong associa-tion between the time of day when sleep begins and the duration of that sleep (Zulley et al 1981); and the time of day and the rapidity with which people can fall asleep. It seems that the only time-band within which people can both fall asleep easily and sleep for 7+ hours (Lavie 1986) is between 10 p.m. and 2 a.m. When sleep is repeatedly curtailed on a succession of nights, symptoms such as fatigue, stress and irritability occur.

Rotating shift patterns appear to produce the greatest problems since there is not time for full adjustment to occur before the next change in sleep–wake scheduling takes over. Permanent night workers suffer fewer ill-effects.

Shiftwork not only affects the workers themselves, but also their partners. Smith & Folkard (1993) found that a sizeable pro-portion of shiftworkers' partners were unhappy with their work patterns, and found that their lives were substantially disrupted by it. While for some, the possibility of working nights may be very convenient, e.g. for young mothers covering child care, for others the disruption has few beneficial effects.

Shiftwork and health

Many individuals are sufficiently resilient that they incur no ill-effects from shiftwork. Others, however, are not so lucky. The most rapidly apparent problems occurring as a result of night work are sleep disruption, fatigue, stress and irritability. There are other, more long-term health risks which may result in more serious problems such as cardiovascular disease, gastrointestinal disorders and psychiatric disorders.

The greater the time spent working nights, the greater the risk of heart disease (Waterhouse et al 1992), possibly due to disturbances in normal physiology. This effect persists even when the influence of smoking is taken into account. Research findings vary, but several have shown an increase in the incidence of anxiety and depression (e.g. Costa et al 1981), which themselves may be linked to heart disease.

Meal times are zeitgebers for certain circadian rhythms, and the loss of appetite which commonly coincides with night-shift work can increase physiological desynchronisation. Disrupted eating and sleeping patterns can result in constipation, indigestion, flatulence and an increased likelihood of developing stomach ulcers (Vener et al 1989). The content as well as the timing of meals may change, with more carbohydrate-based snacks being eaten.

It has been suggested that sufferers of certain health problems should be exempted from working nights (Koller 1989). These conditions include:

• gastrointestinal disorders such as stomach ulcers
• diabetes, because of the need for regular medication and meal times
• epilepsy, since sleep deficits increase the likelihood of seizure
• chronic heart disease
• severe neurotic disorders.

It is not only physical health which can suffer. Even moderate changes in the timing of the sleep–wake cycle may have profound effects on subsequent mood. In healthy young subjects (like the majority of nurses), subjective mood is influenced by interactions of circadian phase and the length of prior wakefulness (Boivin et al 1997).

Shiftwork and performance

When partial sleep deprivation is accrued over several nights, performance and therefore safety may be affected. In the early hours of the morning, alertness and the ability to perform are normally at their lowest. Partial sleep deprivation combined with this natural trough can then result in impaired judgement. Although the kinds of tasks most affected are those requiring vigilance, and repetitive actions, nurses may be prone to more errors in terms of calculating drug dosages, or observing electrocardiogram (ECG) monitors accurately.

It is therefore important for night-shift workers to gain enough sleep to ensure safe practice and personal well-being and health. Some possible strategies for minimising the ill-effects of night-shift work are shown in Table 11.5.

Certain patterns of night working seem better than others, e.g. permanent night shifts seem to produce less personal disruption than rotating shift patterns.

Those working rotating shifts may use hypnotic drugs such as temazepam to help them sleep during the day. This may be successful in the short term, but would be ill-advised for long-term use (see Ch. 10). The hormone melatonin acts as a synchroniser

Table 11.5 Minimising the impact of night-shift work

Area of concern	Action
Timing of sleep	Try to sleep straight after a first night shift, rather than trying to take extra sleep in the latter part of the previous day
	For subsequent nights, try to sleep immediately after the shift; if this is not possible, try immediately after lunchtime (in the post-lunch circadian dip)
	If you take a break during the night shift, a short nap can ease fatigue
Sleeping environment	Find a dark, quiet and comfortable place to sleep. Use earplugs if necessary
	Let friends and relatives know you will be sleeping, to minimise disturbance from the phone, or impromptu visits
	A small alcoholic drink before settling may hasten the onset of sleep (larger amounts will disturb sleep later on)
Regular habits	Eat freshly prepared meals regularly, and avoid nibbling junk food throughout shifts
	Take some exercise on a regular basis, preferably after daytime sleep
	Structure domestic tasks such as shopping, to help maintain a routine

of circadian rhythms and has been shown to improve problems related to sleep when given at bedtime. It has been highly successful in alleviating jet lag. It produces increased alertness during working hours, especially during the early morning. However, effects on performance are not clear (Folkard et al 1993). Currently melatonin is unavailable in the UK, although it can be bought over the counter in many countries.

Delaying shift systems seem easier to adjust to than advancing ones (Barton & Folkard 1993). This is because it is easier to adjust to a longer day – it is easier to maintain wakefulness for longer than normal, than to attempt to sleep before the usual sleeping time.

To conclude, there are many predictable social and physiological events which can influence sleep. Special 'at-risk' groups have been identified in this chapter. Midwives and health visitors have an important role in the sleep of pregnant women and infants respectively. Hospital and community-based nurses have a great deal of contact with the group at highest risk of sleep problems, that is, elderly people. The ability to differentiate between avoidable and unavoidable changes in sleep should provide all nurses with the ability to help these groups (and in some cases themselves) manage their sleep.

REFERENCES

Agnew H W, Webb W B, Williams R L 1996 The first night effect: an EEG study of sleep. Psychophysiology 12: 412–415
Allen S R, Seiler W O, Stähelen H B, Speigel R 1987 Seventy two hour polygraphic and behavioral recordings of wakefulness and sleep in a hospital geriatric unit: comparison between demented and non-demented patients. Sleep 10: 143–159
Ancoli-Israel S, Parker L, Sinaee R, Fell R L, Kripke D F 1989 Sleep fragmentation in patients from a nursing home. Journal of Gerontology: Medical Sciences 44: 18–21
Anders T, Keener M 1985 Developmental course of night time sleep–wake patterns in full-term and premature infants during the first year of life sleep 8(3): 173–192
Barton J, Folkard S 1993 Advancing versus delaying shift systems. Ergonomics 36(1–3): 59–64
Bax M C O 1980 Sleep disturbances in the young child. British Medical Journal 280: 1177–1179
Bliwise D 1993 Sleep in normal ageing and dementia. Sleep 16: 40–81
Boivin D B, Czeisler C A, Dijk D J et al 1997 Complex interaction of the sleep–wake cycle and circadian phase modulates mood in healthy subjects. Archives of General Psychiatry 54(2): 145–152

Brocklehurst J C, Fry J, Griffiths L L, Kalton G 1971 Dysuria in old age. Journal of the American Geriatrics Society 19: 582–592

Carskaden M A, Dement W C 1987 Sleepiness in the normal adolescent. In: Guilleminault C (Ed) Sleep and its disorders in children. Raven Press, New York

Carty E M, Bradley C, Winslow W 1996 Women's perceptions of fatigue during pregnancy and postpartum: the impact of length of hospital stay. Clinical Nursing Research 5(1): 67–80

Coble P A, Kupfer D J, Reynolds C F, Houck P 1987 EEG sleep of healthy children 6 to 12 years of age. In: Guilleminault C (ed) Sleep and its disorders in children. Raven Press, New York, pp 32–33

Costa G, Apostoli P, D'Andrea F, Gaffuri E 1981 Gastrointestinal and neurotic disorders in textile shift workers. In: Reinberg A, Vieux N, Andlauer P (eds) Night and shift work: biological and social aspects. Pergamon, Oxford

Crawford W, Bennet R, Hewitt K 1989 Sleep problems in pre-school children. Health Visitor 62: 79–81

Dew M A, Reynolds C F, Monk T H et al 1994 Psychosocial correlates and sequelae of electroencephalographic sleep in healthy elders. Journal of Gerontology: Psychological Sciences 49: 8–18

Entwisle D, Doering S 1981 The first birth: a family turning point. Johns Hopkins University Press, Baltimore

Erlik Y, Tataryn I V, Meldrum D R, Lomax P, Bajorek J G, Judd H L 1981 Association of waking episodes with menopausal hot flushes. Journal of the American Medical Association 245(17): 1741–1744

Evans M L, Dick M J, Clark A S 1995 Sleep during the week before labor: relationships to labor outcomes. Clinical Nursing Research 4(3): 238–249

Fast A, Hertz G 1992 Nocturnal low back pain in pregnancy: polysomnographic correlates. American Journal of Reproductive Immunology 28(3–4): 251–253

Fleming P J, Blair P S, Bacon C et al 1996 Environment of infants during sleep and risk of the sudden infant death syndrome: results of 1993–5 case-control study for confidential inquiry into still births and deaths in infancy. British Medical Journal 313(7051): 191–195

Folkard S, Arendt J, Clark M 1993 Can melatonin improve shift workers' tolerance of the night shift? Some preliminary findings. Chronobiology International 10(5): 315–320

Galbraith L, Hewitt K, Pritchard L 1993 Behavioural treatment for sleep disturbance. Health Visitor 66(5): 169–171

Gilhooly M 1984 The social dimensions of senile dementia. In: Hanley I, Hodge J (eds) Psychological approaches to the care of the elderly. Croom Helm, London, pp 88–135

Gilleard C J 1986 Living with dementia. Croom Helm, London

Gislason T, Almqvist M 1987 Somatic diseases and sleep complaints. Acta Medica Scandanavica 221: 475–481

Habte-Gabr E, Wallace R B, Colsher P L, Hulbert J R, White L R, Smith I M 1991 Sleep patterns in rural elders: demographic, health and psychobehavioural correlates. Journal of Clinical Epidemiology 44: 5–13

Hertz G, Fast A, Feinsilver S H, Albertario C L, Schulman H, Fein A M 1992 Sleep in normal late pregnancy. Sleep 15(3): 246–251

Hinchcliffe A C, Hyman I, Blizard B, Livingston G 1992 The impact on carers of behavioural difficulties in dementia: a pilot study on management. International Journal of Geriatric Psychiatry 7: 579–583

Jenkins S 1980 Behaviour problems in young children. Health Visitor 53: 463–465

Jones D P H, Verduyn C M 1983 Behavioural management of sleep problems. Archives of Disease in Childhood 58: 442–444

Kerr S M, Jowett S A, Smith L N 1996 Preventing sleep problems in infants: a randomized controlled trial. Journal of Advanced Nursing 24: 938–942

Koller M 1989 Preventive health measures for shiftworkers. In: Wallace M (ed) Managing shiftwork. Brain Behaviour Research Institute, 17–24 La Trobe University, Bundoora, Australia

Lavie P 1986 Ultrashort sleep–waking schedule. 'Gates' and 'forbidden zones' for sleep. Electroencephalography and Clinical Neurophysiology 63: 414–425

Lee K A, DeJoseph J F 1992 Sleep disturbances, vitality and fatigue among a select group of employed childbearing women. Birth 19(4): 208–213

Lentz M J, Killien M G 1991 Are you sleeping? Sleep patterns during postpartum hospitalization. Journal of Perinatal and Neonatal Nursing 4(4): 30–38

Middelcoop H A M, Kerkhof G A, Smilde-Van Den Doel D A, Ligthart G J, Kamphuisen H A C 1994 Sleep and ageing: the effects of institutionalisation on subjective and objective characteristics of sleep. Age and Ageing 23: 411–417

Monk T H, Reynolds C F, Machen M A Kupfer D J 1992 Daily social rhythms in the elderly and their relationship to objectively recorded sleep. Sleep 15: 322–329

Morgan K 1987 Sleep and Ageing. Croomhelm, Beckenham

Morgan K 1990 Hypnotics in the elderly: what cause for concern? Drugs 40: 688–696

Morgan K 1996 Mental health factors in late-life insomnia. Reviews in Clinical Gerontology 6: 75–83

Mosko S, Richard C, McKenna J 1997 Maternal Sleep and arousals during bed sharing with infants. Sleep 20(2): 142–150

Ottaviano S, Gianolti F, Cortesi F, Brini O, Ottaviano C 1996 Sleep characteristics in healthy children from birth to 6 years of age in the urban area of Rome. Sleep 19(1): 1–3

Pollack C P, Perlick D 1991 Sleep problems and institutionalization of the elderly. Journal of Geriatric Psychiatry and Neurology 15: 123–135

Preston F S 1973 Further sleep problems in airline pilots on world-wide schedules. Aerospace Medicine 44: 775–782

Prinz P N, Peskind E R, Vitaliano P P et al 1982 Changes in the sleep and waking EEGs of non-demented and demented elderly subjects 30: 86–93

Reynolds C F, Kupfer D J, Taska L S, Hoch C C, Sewitch D E, Spiker D G 1985 Sleep of healthy seniors: a revisit. Sleep 8: 20–29

Richman N, Stevenson J E, Graham P J 1975 Prevalence of behaviour problems in 3 year old children: an epidemiological study in a London Borough. Journal of Child Psychology and Psychiatry 16: 277–287

Rutenfranz J, Haider M, Koller M 1985 Occupational health measures for nightworkers and shiftworkers. In: Folkard S, Monk T H (eds) Hours of work – temporal factors in work scheduling. Wiley, New York

Sadeh A, Dark I, Vohr B R 1996 Newborns' sleep–wake patterns: the role of maternal, delivery and infant factors. Early Human Development 44(2): 113–126

Sadler S 1994 Sleep: what is normal at six months? Professional Care of Mother and Child 4(6): 166–167

Scharf M B, Kales A, Bixler E O 1975 Readaptation to the sleep laboratory in insomniac subjects. Psychophysiology 12: 412–415

Shaver J, Goblin E, Leutz M, Lee K 1988 Sleep Patterns and stability in peri-menopausal Women. Sleep 11(6): 556–561

Smith L, Folkard S 1993 The perceptions and feelings of shiftworkers' partners. Ergonomics 36(103): 299–305

Spelten E, Barton J, Folkard S 1993 Have we underestimated shiftworkers' problems? Evidence from a 'reminiscence' study. Ergonomics 36(1–3): 307–312

Suzuki S, Dennerstein L, Greenwood K M, Armstrong S M, Satohisa E 1994 Sleeping patterns during pregnancy in Japanese Women. Journal of Psychosomatic Obstetrics and Gynaecology 15(1): 19–26

Thomas R 1997 Clinical update. Nocturnal enuresis: a private agony. Health Visitor 70(1): 34–35

Vener K J, Szabo S, Moore J G 1989 The effect of shift work on gastrointestinal (GI) function: a review. Chronobiologia 16: 421–439

Walsh J K, Moss K L, Sugarman J 1994 Insomnia in adult psychiatric disorders. In: Kryger M H, Roth T, Dement W C (eds) Principles and practice of sleep medicine. W B Saunders, Philadelphia

Waters M A, Lee K A 1996 Differences between primigravidae and multigravidae mothers in sleep disturbances, fatigue, and functional status. Journal of Nurse-Midwifery 41(5): 364–367

Waterhouse J M, Folkard S, Minors D S (1992) Shiftwork, Health and Safety. An overview of the scientific literature 1978–1990. HMSO, London

Webb W B 1981 Sleep stage responses of older and younger subjects after sleep deprivation. Electroencephalography and Clinical Neurophysiology 52: 368–371

Wessel M A, Cobb J C, Jackson E B, Harris G S, Detwiler A C 1954 Paroxysmal fussing in infancy, sometimes called 'colic'. Pediatrics 14: 421–434

Williams R L, Karacan I, Hursch C 1974 EEG of human sleep. Wiley, New York

Willinger M, Hoffman H J, Hartford R B 1994 Infant sleep position and risk for sudden infant death syndrome: report of meeting held January 13 and 14, 1994, National Institutes of Health, Bethesda, MD. Pediatrics 93(5): 814–819

Wolfson A, Lacks P, Futterman A 1992 Effects of parent training on infant sleeping patterns, parents' stress, and perceived parental competence. Journal of Consulting and Clinical Psychology 60(1): 41–48

Woodward S, Freedman R R 1994 The thermoregulatory effects of menopausal hot flushes on sleep. Sleep 17(6): 497–501

Zulley J, Wever R A, Aschoff J 1981 The dependence of onset and duration of sleep on the circadian rhythm of rectal temperature. Pflugers Archiv. European Journal of Physiology 391: 314–318

Sleep management within special environments

Learning outcomes

This chapter examines some of the causes and consequences of sleep disturbance within institutional settings, and considers the implications of such disturbance for nursing practice. On completing this chapter you should be able to:

- name six common causes of sleep disturbance in hospital
- describe three physiological effects of disturbed sleep in hospital
- describe three psychological consequences of disturbed sleep in hospitals
- identify three practical strategies to minimise sleep disturbances in hospital patients.

INTRODUCTION

It seems appropriate to begin this chapter with a quote from the Vice-Chair of the British Patients Association: 'Patients come in all shapes and sizes and their opinions are as diverse. But there is one thing about which they are almost unanimous; that it's very difficult to get a good night's sleep in hospital' (Marcus 1995).

For most people, admission to hospital disrupts normal patterns of rest and activity. In general, the times of settling down at night and morning waking are earlier than at home; the duration of their sleep is reduced; more night-time awakenings occur; and subjective sleep quality tends to decline. It is also well recognised in contemporary sleep research that environmental novelty (such as the first night in the electroencephalogram (EEG) laboratory) results in sleep which is shorter, lighter, and more broken, a phenomenon originally described as the 'first night effect' (Agnew et al 1966, Scharf et al 1975). There is no reason to suppose that such phenomena do not initially accompany institutional admissions. Overall, then, the experience of hospital admission may, for many, produce some degree of situational insomnia and sleep deprivation, which may have implications for recovery from illness or surgery. In this chapter, evidence is presented concerning: the ill-effects resulting from poor sleep; the difficulties of sleeping in hospital; and the factors which cause the greatest sleep problems for inpatients. Practical suggestions are then made as to how ward nurses might intervene both to help patients during hospitalisation, and prevent the development of longer-term problems.

SLEEP AND SLEEP DEPRIVATION
Physiological effects of sleep deprivation

Since the beginning of the 20th century, researchers have investigated the nature and purpose of sleep using the experimental paradigm of sleep deprivation, where volunteers or laboratory animals are deliberately prevented from going to sleep. While a comprehensive theory of sleep function (i.e. what sleep is *for*) that satisfies all researchers remains elusive, a considerable literature now exists describing the physiological and psychological consequences of sleeplessness. This literature has been thoroughly reviewed by Horne (1988), who concluded that while the cerebral cortex appears to show the greatest need for sleep, sustained sleep deprivation produces a generalised physiological 'slowing up'. When people are *totally* sleep deprived (i.e. prevented from getting *any* sleep), their subsequent 'recovery' sleep (see Ch. 7) appears to compensate for some of the loss. Thus, recovery sleep tends to be longer, with proportionally higher levels of slow wave sleep (SWS) (i.e. stages 3 and 4) than 'normal' sleep. Since stages 1, 2 and rapid eye movement (REM) show less or no recovery, this evidence strongly suggests that SWS is the component of sleep which is of greatest importance to our functioning. *Partial* sleep deprivation is, however, more likely in general wards and it seems that only when sleep is reduced below 3 hours, is a substantial loss of SWS observed (see Horne 1988).

Sleep and tissue restoration

It has long been thought that sleep disturbance impairs tissue restoration (e.g. Adam & Oswald 1983), with recent research indicating that SWS coincides with peak anabolic (tissue-building) processes (Shapiro & Flanigan 1993). Most human growth hormone (hGH) is also secreted during the first 3 hours of sleep, and is associated with the main period of SWS (Gronfier et al 1996). In addition, there is evidence that the duration of SWS is higher when the body has a greater need for growth (for example, during adolescence, pregnancy, after exercise and after sleep loss).

Sleep and body temperature

SWS also appears to conserve energy by downregulating body temperature and metabolic rate (Berger & Phillips 1995). Metabolic rate is reduced by 5–25% during the night. Many hospital patients need to conserve energy for the simple reason that they are (usually temporarily) undernourished. Patients are often starved for surgery or other procedures; or they may have lost their appetite or be unable to eat without assistance. This state of starvation depletes energy resources, and may contribute to the fatigue often experienced by inpatients. SWS may therefore exert a protective effect under these circumstances. Starvation appears to be accompanied by a significant rise in SWS and a fall in REM, supporting this idea (MacFadyen et al 1973).

Sleep deprivation also tends to lower core body temperature slightly, by 0.3–0.4°C. This magnitude of fall is statistically significant, but it has no obvious clinical significance unless a patient has an unusually high or low temperature anyway. It might increase subjective feelings of cold, it might temporarily mask an infection by delaying the detection of pyrexia, or it may exaggerate hypothermia. In such cases, thermoregulatory mechanisms are not actually impaired, it is simply that body temperature is reset at a lower level than normal.

Sleep and immune function

The evidence also suggests that sleep quality has direct implications for immune function. The onset of SWS coincides with greater immunological activity – including the lymphocyte responses to antigens and natural killer cell activity (Moldofsky et al 1989). Compromised immunity may present a particular problem for some hospital patients, since they are usually subject to various stresses which result in raised cortisol levels. Cortisol itself dampens down the immune response. This is obviously undesirable, given the increased likelihood of picking up infections during a hospital stay.

Sleep and cerebral recovery

Horne's (1988) detailed review of the literature concluded that sleep is essential for the recovery and restitution of neural and related tissues. It appears that the brain itself cannot maintain long periods of excitation (as during wakefulness or REM sleep) so it alternates these states with SWS for homeostatic reasons. During SWS, the deeper layer of the cerebral cortex partially shuts down. This may allow it to recover from the 'wear and tear' caused by brain activity during wakefulness and REM. Horne emphasised that this 'cerebral impairment is not to be viewed as brain damage, but as a reversible state, analogous to the impairment and recovery of muscle after exercise' (1988, p. 46). Unlike muscle, however, brain tissue only recovers during sleep, not through rest alone.

Psychological effects of sleep deprivation

In addition to having a generally detrimental impact on physiological functioning, sleep deprivation can also influence how we feel, and the efficiency of our everyday activities. These effects, the psychological consequences of partial or total sleep deprivation, can have both indirect and direct implications for patient well-being.

Vigilance

Vigilance, the ability to sustain attention and concentrate, is markedly reduced after one night's total sleep deprivation. After three or more nights of no sleep, mental processes are markedly slowed, and there may be frequent loss of a train of thought, or even incoherent thoughts and speech. Most at risk are monotonous tasks (like car driving) where the need to maintain alertness is paramount. Those who are sleep deprived also tend to lose track of time.

Mind and mood

Extended total sleep deprivation can result in visual misperceptions, temporal disorientation and cognitive disorganisation. These tend to worsen as the duration of sleep deprivation gets longer. Mood changes (such as irritability and mania), reduced motivation, confusion and (rarely) paranoia may also occur. All of these are potentially detrimental to recovery from illness or surgery, since they may reduce the willingness or the ability of patients to undertake activities of daily living, such as taking adequate fluids or mobilising. The relative importance a patient attaches to sleep, and its relationship to recovery in hospital, should also be recognised here. Patients frequently hold beliefs that sleep can have a positive influence on health and healing, the ability to cope and the experience of pain, as the examples provided in Table 12.1 demonstrate.

Table 12.1 The beliefs of hospital patients about their sleep (Closs 1992b)

Effects of sleep	Patients' comments
Sleep and healing	'... sleep is the best healer in the world. You know it's going to take longer to get better if you can't get your sleep.'
	'Sleep is the best medicine–better than a feed when you're ill. If you're sleeping, you're getting better the whole time.'
	'You've got to get a good sleep before you get anything else. You feel fresh and don't get crabby, you can deal with the pain and everything else, and it speeds up your recovery.'
Sleep and coping	'[sleep] is essential–you can't cope with anything unless you've slept.'
	'You're not so well able to cope if you're tired, you have a good attitude if you're rested.'
	'Even an hour's sound sleep in the middle of the day can raise spirits.'
Sleep and pain	'If you're tired and in pain you want to give up quicker. You could have shot me yesterday for all I cared.'
	'When you're tired and anxious it builds up the level of pain.'
	'If you've slept well the pain isn't as bad a blow when you awaken. If you don't sleep you wonder when it'll ever end. It's a vicious circle.'
	'The pain is more nagging and it's harder to put up with if you're tired.'

SLEEP DISTURBANCE IN HOSPITALS

While there are numerous sources of sleep disruption within hospital settings, not all are present in all wards. Here we consider evidence of some of the more common causes of sleeplessness, and how these might be dealt with.

By far, the most commonly cited cause of sleep disturbance in hospital is noise. In acute areas such as ICU and surgical wards, pain is a major cause. In addition to these, both necessary and unnecessary nursing and medical care disturb patients at night. Anxiety is a problem for many and there are frequent complaints that beds are uncomfortable and that the environment is too hot, too cold or too brightly lit. Sleeping may be more difficult because of changes in normal routines such as earlier bedtimes and waking, and some patients have difficulty sleeping simply because they are in a strange environment. All of these causes of sleep disturbance have been cited in various studies (Clapin-French 1986, Closs 1992a, Cox 1992, Dodds 1980, Hilton 1976, Johns et al 1974, Lentz & Killien 1991, Murphy et al 1977, Ogilvie 1980, Pacini & Fitzpatrick 1982, Reimer 1987, Royal Commission on the NHS 1978, Southwell & Wistow 1995, Stead 1985, Yinnon et al 1992).

Sleep disruption in general wards

Different researchers have used different approaches to the assessment of sleep disruption, so studies are not always comparable one with another. Several researchers have provided objective evidence of the extent of sleep disruption suffered by hospital inpatients by monitoring with all-night polysomnography (see Ch. 1). Subjective methods, namely observation of patients sleeping, or patients' own reports, have also been used in order to assess the causes and extent of sleep disruptions of less acutely ill patients. Some of the major studies which have measured frequency of sleep disturbance and the duration of night-time sleep are shown in Tables 12.2 and 12.3.

In addition, the survey by the Royal Commission on the National Health Service (1978) indicated that more than a quarter of the 699 patients interviewed were generally disturbed during the night, although no details were given. A smaller study of sleep patterns in 50 low-dependency patients using an interview

Table 12.2 Number of sleep disturbances experienced by hospital patients; a summary of research studies

Author	Sample	No. of nocturnal sleep disruptions
Walker (1972)	Four cardiotomy patients on their first postoperative night	7 per hour (observed)
Woods (1972)	Four cardiotomy patients on their first postoperative night	Mean = 59.5 (observed)
Kavey & Altschuler (1979)	10 herniorrhaphy patients	Preoperative mean = 4.9 (polygraph) First postoperative night mean = 12.5 Third postoperative night mean = 8.5
Closs (1988)	200 patients on surgical and ENT wards	Mean = 2.3 (reported by patient)
Fontaine (1989)	20 trauma patients	32 (polygraph)
Knill et al (1990)	12 abdominal surgery patients	Preoperative mean = 9 (polygraph) First postoperative night mean = 21 Third postoperative night mean = 12
Lentz & Killien (1991)	34 postpartum mothers	Mode 3–4 (reported by mothers)
Closs (1992a)	100 abdominal surgery patients, third postoperative night	Mean = 3.3 (reported by patients)
Rosenberg et al (1994)	10 abdominal surgery patients	Preoperative median = 18 (polygraph) First postoperative night median = 21 Second postoperative night median = 16
Sheely (1996)	50 oncology patients	Mean 15.7 (observed)

schedule showed that 76% felt that they accrued a sleep deficit over three nights compared with sleep at home. 44% of these sustained a 4-hour deficit and 18% more than a 6-hour deficit (Carter, unpublished work, 1984). Southwell & Wistow (1995) found that two-thirds of patients on medical, surgical, psychiatric and care of the elderly wards were disturbed at night. On average, these patients reported 3.7 different causes of disturbance, mainly concerned with different types of noise.

It is clear from these findings that those who are undergoing more acute hospital care have the shortest, most disturbed sleep. However, these reductions in sleep need to be considered in more

Table 12.3 Duration of night-time sleep in hospital: a summary of research studies

Author	Sample	Duration of sleep
Johns et al (1974)	Five cardiac or abdominal surgery patients	1–4 hours in first 24 hours after surgery (polygraph)
Orr & Stahl (1977)	Nine cardiac or thoracic, surgery patients	Eight out of nine had no sleep on first postoperative night (polygraph)
Hilton (1976)	10 patients in respiratory ICU	2.6 hours (polygraph)
Kavey & Altschuler (1979)	10 herniorrhaphy patients	Preoperative mean = 6.1 hours (polygraph) First postoperative night mean = 6.4 hours Third postoperative night mean = 6.2 hours
Floyd (1984)	35 psychiatric inpatients	7.6–8.2 hours (reported)
Aurell & Elmqvist (1985)	Nine non-cardiac postoperative patients, first postoperative night in ICU	Mean of 1 h 51 min. Five patients had no sleep (polygraph)
Closs (1988)	200 patients on surgical or ENT wards	5.4 hours (reported)
Fontains (1989)	20 trauma patients	4.2 hours (polygraph)
Knill et al (1990)	12 abdominal surgery patients	Preoperative mean = 5.45 (polygraph) First postoperative night mean = 5.3 hours Third postoperative night mean = 5.5 hours
Closs (1992a)	100 abdominal surgery patients, third postoperative night	5.8 hours (reported)
Lane & Fontaine (1992)	Nine children, mean age, 4.7 years in paediatric ICU	4.7 hours (observed)
Rosenberg et al (1994)	10 abdominal surgery	Preoperative median = 5.5 (polygraph) First postoperative night median = 5.8 hours Third postoperative night median = 5.6 hours
Closs et al (1998)	417 orthopaedic patients	Second postoperative night mean = 4.8 hours (reported)

detail. Since different stages of sleep make different contributions to restoration, their loss is of varying significance. In addition, the possibility of compensatory napping during the day may be important but has rarely been reported.

CAUSES OF SLEEP DISTURBANCE IN HOSPITALS

Noise

Without doubt, the worst problem as far as most patients are concerned is the noise level in hospital. There are many different causes of noise, some within and some beyond the control of the nurse, but at night, all are undesirable and cause more distress than is commonly realised. This has been clearly expressed by Augarde (1995) a nurse who, after being a patient herself, commented: 'I found the problem of night-time noise seriously distressing and disruptive to my well-being and recovery ....What may seem a trivial issue remains one of the most memorably distressing features of an unpleasant illness experience. It appears to be remembered likewise by many other ex-hospital patients I have spoken to.'

The International Noise Council (see Grumet 1993) recommend that noise levels in acute areas of hospitals should be limited to 45 A-weighted decibels (dB(A)) during the daytime, 40 dB(A) in the evening and 20 dB(A) at night. What does this mean? First of all, A-weighted decibels are from a scale which filters out lower frequency sounds and emphasises higher frequency ones, in a way which approximates to the human range of hearing. How loud is a decibel? 20 dB(A) is the loudness of a whisper, or the ticking of a watch. 40–50 dB(A) is equivalent to light traffic, or a quiet hospital environment; intermediate is 50–60 dB(A), as loud as a telephone; and 60–70 dB(A) is unacceptably noisy. (The decibel scale is not linear; for each increase of 10 decibels there is an approximate doubling of the subjective perception of the loudness of a sound.)

According to Grumet (1993), ambient noise levels in most modern hospitals in the USA range from 50–70 dB(A) with occasional bursts of louder noise. A British study of psychiatric, general, medical and acute admitting wards showed average noise levels of between 49 and 68 dB(A) (Soutar & Wilson 1986). The quietest area was the psychiatric ward and the noisiest were the general and acute medical wards. There was no apparent difference between the levels of noise during the day and the night. A more recent study of noise in an intensive care unit (ICU) found a large number of sound peaks above 80 dB(A) at night and this was closely associated with the number of arousals from sleep (Aaron et al 1996).

The amount of noise needed to wake people up depends on several things, for example, what stage of sleep they are in, their age and their sex. A 36 dB(A) noise for 3 minutes will wake about half of people in stage 2 sleep, while 83 dB(A) is needed to wake up those in SWS. Older people are more sensitive to the effects of noise than younger ones, even though many of them may have hearing difficulties. A 20-year-old is half as likely to be disturbed by a given noise than someone who is 70.

The effects of noise on hospital patients

Noises elicit both physiological and psychological responses in all of us. For hospital patients, they may act as yet another stressor. The auditory nerves influence those areas of the brain concerned with arousal and attention, particularly the ascending reticular activating system and the thalamus. Loud noises cause both immediate and slightly delayed responses. They produce an immediate response from the nervous system and voluntary musculature, the 'startle' response. This usually includes blinking and/or grimacing.

Secondary responses then occur, including reduced motility of the smooth muscle of the gut, decreased secretions from the stomach and salivary glands, desynchronisation of the EEG, peripheral vasoconstriction, slowed breathing, rapid pulse and hyperreflexia. Noise can raise the levels of the vasoconstrictor angiotensin II, cholesterol and triglycerides. The adrenal glands produce increased adrenaline and noradrenaline following noisy stimuli; a response which may be greatly exaggerated in anxious patients. This may lead to high levels of hydroxycorticosteroids in the blood. The physiological arousal due to these endocrine responses occurs directly after the noise stimulus, and may continue for up to 2 hours (particularly undesirable for someone who has been admitted following, say, myocardial infarction).

These responses are most noticeable in patients who wake up because of noise, or who were already awake. However, being asleep does not prevent the body from responding to noises. The EEG of sleeping patients shows changes, even if the individuals do not wake up fully. There may be signs of brief arousals and shifts to lighter stages of sleep. Other changes also occur, such as vasoconstriction and increased heart rate. But it is not just the ill who are disturbed by noise in hospitals. Noise also has an adverse effect on newborn infants. Two studies which compared babies in normal hospital conditions with babies in a quiet environment showed that those exposed to quieter conditions slept for longer, cried less, fed more quickly and gained more weight (Keefe 1987, Mann et al 1986).

Noisy environments can affect wakeful behaviour, too. Exposure to constant loud noise may produce annoyance and aggression in certain individuals. Concentration may be impaired, and cognitive processes impeded. There have been few studies of the effect of noise in hospitals on inpatients, although one (Fife & Rappaport 1976) found that there was a positive correlation between the amount of noise and length of stay for surgical patients. Interestingly, Bailey (1981) found that noise was the most important reason for patients opting to take hypnotic drugs while in hospital.

Obviously noise is not a problem for everyone – some find it intrusive, others hardly notice. An overview of surveys on noise annoyance suggested that about one-fifth of the population is highly sensitive to noise, while one-quarter is 'unperturbable' (Schultz 1978).

Sources of noise in hospital

Noise in a hospital issues from many sources, both within and outwith wards. In the ward, there is often noisy equipment, such as i.v. alarms, bedpan washers/macerators and telephones. The patients themselves may be noisy, especially if they are confused or in pain. The nursing and medical staff may be noisy, communicating with one another and with patients, and in giving care. Doubtless some of this noise is unavoidable, but there is much that can be reduced with a little thought and care.

Keeping doors closed at night can help to reduce noise in hospital wards. The design of the nurses' station is very important – if it were enclosed in double glazing, the sound of telephones ringing and nurses talking to one another could be better contained. However, speakers would need to be installed inside the station to transmit sound from the ward. Obviously it would be important for nurses to be able to hear if patients called out. Where this is not possible, nurses and other staff should be ever mindful of how loudly they are speaking, and make all efforts to keep noise to a minimum. Talking to patients is unavoidable, and frequently desirable at night, but should be done as quietly as possible.

Noisy equipment also presents problems. Radios and televisions should only be used with headsets after lights out, and telephones should have their volume turned down where possible. Some telephones have a graduated ring, which starts quietly and gradually becomes louder, which is less disturbing for those trying to sleep. The type of pagers which vibrate rather than bleep are preferable for contacting on-call staff at night.

A perennial cause for complaint is the noise made by doctors and nurses simply walking around. Leather-soled shoes can be very noisy, and squeaky shoes, or shoes with loose buckles are also intrusive. Lace-up shoes with quiet soles have long been advocated as suitable for hospital staff, yet this kind of footwear is still not mandatory in all hospitals.

Alarms on clinical equipment should be kept as quiet as possible – the beeping of i.v. pump alarms can be extremely annoying. At night, flashing lights to indicate that the alarm has been set off would be much less intrusive. They should be pointed away from the patients' eyes, but be obvious to night staff.

In some cases, patients with no history of confusion become severely confused within the first 5 days following surgery. This kind of delirium is most common among elderly people. These patients require special attention, and may need to be moved out of the main ward into a single room to prevent them from disturbing other patients. In some cases, cot-sides may be needed to prevent them from falling out of bed, and others may require sedation.

Despite the consistent evidence indicating that hospitals are noisy places, Southwell & Wistow (1995) found discrepancies between nurses' and patients' reports of sleep disturbance. More nurses reported noise due to treatments, commodes/bedpans, toilets flushing and nurses talking to patients. More patients reported noise outside the ward, emergencies, patients making a noise, nurses' shoes and nurses talking to one another. So there appears to be some kind of qualitative difference between the perceptions of patients and nurses. Nurses were more aware of noise related to their work. They were less aware of noises coming from outside the ward, presumably because they were more used to them. Fewer nurses reported noise from emergencies, perhaps because they were unaware of noise while dealing with urgent situations. Finally, nurses were largely unaware of their own noisy shoes.

Evidently, then, staff and patients have rather different perceptions of noise at night. A first step in reducing noise, therefore, might be to increase awareness of the problems among night staff. Reducing environmental noise should then be a priority. Another option is to mask sudden noises by providing other constant sounds, such as that of an electric fan. A trial undertaken by Williamson (1992) showed that taped ocean sounds (white noise) significantly improved sleep patterns in a study of 60 postoperative patients.

Pain and discomfort

After noise, pain is probably the second greatest cause of disturbed sleep, particularly for postoperative and other acutely ill patients. Again, this has been expressed clearly by an ex-patient, on this occasion a doctor, writing to *The Lancet* after a spell in hospital: 'my fellow doctors *must* be enlightened ... during the dreadful nights you face the pain, and the horrors brought by fever and half-sleep, alone. It cannot be described' (Freed 1975).

More recently, a report from the Royal College of Surgeons and the College of Anaesthetists (1990) summarised research which showed consistently poor management of postoperative pain in hospitals. Many patients also suffer from chronic pain, such as that caused by arthritis, both at home and in hospital. However, all pain sufferers require careful assessment and treatment of their pain if they are to get the best possible sleep. Pain often seems worse at night owing to the lack of distractions. During the day, there is constant activity in most wards, with nursing observations, doctors' rounds, meal times, visitors and so on. This has the useful side-effect of distracting patients from their pain and reducing their perception of it. Pain can cause muscular tension and agitation, each of which can worsen pain, creating a vicious circle. Relaxation techniques (see Ch. 8) may be effective in breaking this circle and reducing the pain.

Chronic pain itself may have a circadian rhythm of increasing intensity at night (Glyn et al 1976). For example, gastric secretions increase during REM sleep, worsening dyspepsia and pain from gastric ulcers. Most patients will be aware of their own patterns of pain, and some will have their own ways of accommodating it. The coping strategies used at home, may in some cases be continued in hospital. For example, chronic back pain sufferers may find that careful positioning and support minimises their discomfort during the night. While many people suffer acute pain in hospital, those at greatest risk are obviously those who have been injured and those undergoing surgery or other invasive procedures. Postoperative pain has been associated with the following adverse effects.

Changes in the stress response to injury. Raised blood levels of adrenaline and noradrenaline produce increases in pulse rate and blood pressure; increase in catabolic hormones such as cortisol and adrenocorticotrophic hormone cause tissue breakdown and mobilisation of free fatty acids. This is the opposite of what is required following surgery, when healing processes are needed.

Compromised cardiovascular and pulmonary function. These increases in adrenaline and noradrenaline are likely to produce an adrenergic stress response. This in turn increases the possibility of myocardial ischaemia and reduced tissue perfusion in suscep-tible patients, in particular those with pre-existing cardiovascular and pulmonary disorders.

Reduced mobility. Patients are often understandably reluctant to move because of pain. This produces venous stasis which increases the risk of pressure area damage, deep vein thrombosis and pulmonary embolism.

Anxiety. This is not only an unpleasant subjective experience, it may also have physiological consequences. It may increase blood viscosity, fibrinolysis, platelet aggregation and clotting; it may also enhance the hypothalamic responses characteristic of stress and worsen the subjective perception of pain.

Long-term pain. Poorly managed acute pain may result in unnecessary long-term pain. The physical trauma of injury or surgery can cause two kinds of sensory hypersensitivity: sensitisation of peripheral pain receptors in the skin and internal organs; and central sensitisation of the spinal neurons. Stimuli which normally are not perceived as painful at all, such as gentle pressure, then become noxious. It may be days or weeks before the neurons return to normal functioning (Woolf 1995).

Sleep disturbance. Although it is obviously important to control pain, some analgesics may also have a disruptive impact on sleep. Low doses of morphine, for example, cause a reduction in SWS, while higher doses disrupt virtually all stages of sleep, as well as increasing the number of night-time awakenings (Moote et al 1989). As yet there appears to be no research into postoperative patients, so the effects of morphine on postoperative sleep are not clear. However, even though morphine may disrupt sleep, this must be weighed against the potential ill-effects of pain itself (Rosenberg-Adamsen et al 1996).

As discussed earlier, it is difficult to unpick the relative effects of the unavoidable physiological sequelae of surgery from those responses purely due to postoperative pain. It is important, nevertheless, to ensure that pain is controlled as well as possible in order to permit the best possible sleep under the circumstances. Southwell & Wistow (1995) found that pain was (unsurprisingly) more of a problem on surgical and care of the elderly wards than medical or psychiatric wards. However, they excluded patients with persistent or chronic pain from their sample so they probably underestimated the actual extent of sleep disturbance due to pain.

Surgery and sleep

Surgery and/or the associated anaesthetics have direct physiological consequences which present possible explanations for commonly observed postoperative sleep disruption. In a comprehensive review, Rosenberg-Adamsen et al (1996) concluded that for the first 3 nights or so following surgery, REM sleep tends to be absent while SWS is reduced. By the middle of the first postoperative week, 'rebound' REM sleep ensues, frequently coinciding with reports of vivid nightmares (Knill et al 1990). Sleep usually returns to normal by the end of the first postoperative week (Kavey & Altschuler 1979). These changes are in line with known physiological responses to trauma. For example cortisol, which is produced in response to the stress of surgery, causes a reduction in REM sleep (Fehm et al 1986, Friess et al 1994), while interleukin-1 is released in response to injury, thereby causing fever, which is also associated with decreased REM sleep (Kent et al 1988). A trauma response explanation is also consistent with evidence that both the duration and magnitude of the operation is associated with the degree of subsequent sleep disturbance (Brimacombe & Macfie 1993, Ellis & Dudley 1976).

Other causes of sleep disturbance

There are many other aspects of the hospital environment which have the potential to interfere with normal sleep. These include sleep routines, uncomfortable beds, temperature, light, anxiety and other medical conditions.

Sleep routines

For most people, normal daily routines are changed following hospital admission. In many wards, settling down and waking up times are earlier than at home. If patients wish to read, or take a walk before settling down to sleep, such activities should be encouraged. Various authors have suggested that more flexibility with such routines would be beneficial (Dodds 1980, Southwell & Wistow 1995, Stead 1985). The majority of patients in these studies reported being woken before they were ready. The still prevalent 6 a.m. waking time should be reconsidered, and stopped where feasible, even if this entails pushing back the timetable for the day. It may also be possible to discontinue the early morning drug round, so that drugs are not given on an empty stomach unless clinically essential. Patients also commented on lights out at 10 p.m., even though activity continued until after midnight.

Uncomfortable beds

Uncomfortable hospital beds have been a cause for complaint for at least 20 years. The Royal Commission on the National Health Service (1978) found that almost half of the 699 inpatients they surveyed complained about rubber or plastic draw sheets. Over half of them found the beds too hard. This was confirmed by Closs (1988) and Southwell & Wistow (1995), who had more than twice as many unsolicited complaints about beds and bedding than any other factor. Again, the plastic covers on pillows and mattresses were particularly disliked.

Ambient temperature

Being too hot or too cold can disturb or prevent sleep. However, in large open wards it is difficult to set the environmental temperature to suit everyone. Being too hot is a more common complaint than being too cold. However, elderly people tend to feel the cold more and should be given extra blankets if necessary. Patients often have subjective feelings of cold when they are feverish.

Light

Lights at night may cause disturbance in two different ways. First, they may simply act as disruptive sensory input. Second, light is a zeitgeber (as discussed in Ch. 1). It acts as a synchroniser of circadian rhythms, the major one being, of course, the sleep–wake cycle. Light is a cue for wakefulness, so at night it may prevent normal sleep patterns for many people. Nightlights which are suspended from the ceiling are more of a problem than those located at skirting-board level. For patients who are well enough not to require constant observation, it may be helpful to draw curtains round their bed. Depending on the geography of the ward, this may shade some patients from unwanted light.

Anxiety

The external hospital environment affects sleep, but there are other, more internal responses to being in hospital, such as pain, anxiety and other physiological and psychological responses. Those admitted with acute illnesses will almost certainly be experiencing stress, and the endocrine response to such stress is partly responsible for the subsequent disruption of sleep. The increase in catecholamines released into the blood produces high levels of noradrenergic activity, increasing wakefulness (Hilakivi 1987).

Specific medical conditions

There is a range of conditions commonly seen in hospital patients which may influence their night-time sleep. For example, impaired thyroid activity may result in changes in the duration of sleep; longer in hypothyroidism and shorter in hyperthyroidism. Compromised cardiac or respiratory function may produce symptoms which are at their worst during sleep, such as angina, palpitations, dyspnoea, hypopnoea and worsening of Cheyne—Stokes respiration. Myocardial infarctions often take place during REM sleep and asthma attacks are most common during the second half of the night.

MANAGING SLEEP DISTURBANCE IN HOSPITALS

All the methods for assessing, managing and monitoring sleep problems already covered in this book are relevant in the situations described in this chapter. Not infrequently, however, clinical and institutional circumstances may limit the available options. For example, patients admitted for investigations are frequently anxious and fasting; patients on an open ward will have little choice but to be subject to the prevailing light and temperature conditions. Nevertheless, in combination with good nursing practice, an awareness of the importance of sleep quality, and a familiarity with the approaches already described can at least minimise the impact of what might be termed 'institutional insomnia'.

CONCLUSIONS

It is evident from the available literature that, for a considerable proportion of patients, hospital admission causes disruption of the normal sleep–wake cycle. Factors affecting sleep patterns are of many kinds. Some are experienced subjectively, such as pain and anxiety; and some are a result of the immediate environment, such as noise, type of bed and temperature. It should be possible for nurses to alleviate subjective suffering due to pain and anxiety and to manipulate some aspects of the patient's environment in order to optimise quality and quantity of sleep.

Different strategies are available for changing clinical practices, for example audit and care protocols. For audit to be successful, ward staff should agree together an aspect of patients' sleep or the hospital environment which they would like to improve. For example, admission assessments of sleep. Baseline monitoring of the content of these assessments could be undertaken, followed by discussion and agreement on desirable content. This should be based on a mixture of research-based evidence about what best practice should be, and pragmatic decisions about what is possible and desirable in actual practice. Changes should be made and another period of monitoring undertaken in order to assess the degree of improvement. Similarly, care protocols could be developed in response to local requirements.

In view of the increasing amount of evidence which suggests that sleep enhances recovery, it may be of considerably greater importance than is generally appreciated, that certain patients receive an optimum quantity and quality of sleep, preferably following as closely as possible their normal 'home sleep' patterns. It could be expected that such a provision might promote and even hasten recovery. An evaluation of nursing interventions designed to achieve this would be a worthwhile project. Box 12.1, summarises the main issues involved in improving the sleep of hospital patients.

Box 12.1   Guidelines for managing sleep for hospital patients

Assessment
Assess sleep on admission and on a daily basis. Assess at a level of detail appropriate to the setting and the individual patient. If patients are awake and worrying during the night, give them the opportunity to talk about what is on their mind.

Action
Act on assessments. Use the information from patients to identify the root cause(s) of any sleep difficulties, and take action to deal with these causes. Check on the effectiveness of any action taken by reassessing sleep.

Facilitate individual preferences
Match usual habits as closely as is possible, e.g. allow pre-sleep rituals, timings of sleep, etc., be as much like at home as possible. Allow nightcap or other drink if this does not interfere with treatment. Help into preferred position for sleeping if possible.
  Keep a snack on the bedside locker in case the patient is hungry during the night. Ensure that a drink is easily available. Ensure that patients are warm enough, and not too warm.
  Allow patients to wake when they are ready, if possible. Do not disturb patients for a 6 a.m. medicine round unless essential drugs are to be given.

Minimise noise
Keep the environment as quiet as possible. Make sure that patients have headsets for listening to television or radio. Wear quiet shoes. Speak quietly and only when absolutely necessary in the open ward. Keep doors closed. Use phones and monitoring equipment with flashing lights (pointing away from patients' eyes) rather than alarm buzzers. Keep all patients as comfortable as possible in order to avoid noise due to distressed patients. Replace bleeping pagers with the kind that vibrate. Place noisy patients in single rooms when possible.
  If noise is unavoidable, the introduction of another, constant noise to mask the effects may help. For example, the sound of an electric fan can reduce the disturbing effects of sudden noise. Patients who wish to could be encouraged to use earplugs.

Minimise pain
Keep pain to a minimum. Ensure regular assessment, act on the assessment, and reassess following the action. Educate patients so that they understand that pain is undesirable and often unnecessary – actively encourage them to request analgesia when they require it.

Box 12.1 *(Cont'd)*

Make patients as comfortable as possible
Although hospital beds are generally considered to be uncomfortable,
attempt to make patients as comfortable as possible under local
circumstances. Adjust beds, pillows and bedding to suit individuals.
In particular, do not use plastic draw sheets unless they are absolutely
necessary. If at all possible, replace old plastic mattress covers with more
modern types of semipermeable waterproof cover, which produce less
uncomfortable sweating.

Minimise light
Avoid bright lights, or flashing lights pointing towards patients' eyes
(e.g. on alarms). Some hospital wards have their night lights at
skirting-board level, which is far less intrusive for most people.

Short-term use of hypnotic drugs
Drugs such as temazepam and triazolam may be used judiciously for
acute admissions having short-term difficulty sleeping. These should be
used over approximately 2–3 consecutive nights to improve sleep. They
should not be taken for longer than 5 days, since tolerance may then
neutralise any beneficial effects.

Ensure quality of care
Problem areas, such as noise reduction or effective pain management
may be improved through the use of audit or sleep protocols. Staffing
levels should be adequate during the night. Where patients are in severe
pain, there should always be two qualified nurses available so that
controlled drugs can be checked and given without delay.

REFERENCES

Aaron J N, Carlisle C C, Carskadon M A, Meyer T J, Hill N S, Millman R P 1996
    Environmental noise as a cause of sleep disruption in an intermediate
    respiratory care unit. Sleep 19(9): 707–710
Adam K, Oswald I 1983 Protein synthesis, bodily renewal and the sleep–wake
    cycle. Clinical Science 65: 561–567
Agnew H W, Webb W B, Williams R L 1966 The first night effect: an EEG study
    of sleep. Psychophysiology 12: 412–415
Augarde K 1995 Plea for more silent nights. Nursing Times 91(29): 22
Aurell J, Elmqvist D 1985 Sleep in the surgical intensive care unit: continuous
    polygraphic recording of sleep in nine patients receiving postoperative care.
    British Medical Journal 290: 1029–1032
Bailey H 1981 Sleep and the hospital patient. Research report 1, Department of
    Nursing and Community Health Studies. The Polytechnic of the South Bank,
    London
Berger R J, Phillips N H 1995 Energy conservation and sleep. Behavioural Brain
    Research 69: 65–73
Brimacombe J, Macfie A G 1993 Peri-operative nightmares in surgical patients.
    Anaesthesia 48: 527–529

Clapin-French E 1986 Sleep patterns of aged persons in long-term care facilities. Journal of Advanced Nursing 11: 57–66

Closs S J 1988 A nursing study of sleep on surgical wards. Nursing Research Unit Report, Department of Nursing Studies, University of Edinburgh

Closs S J 1992a Patients' night-time pain, analgesic provision and sleep after surgery. International Journal of Nursing Studies 29(4): 381–392

Closs S J 1992b Post-operative patients' views of sleep, pain and recovery. Journal of Clinical Nursing 1: 83–88

Closs S J, Gardiner E, Briggs M 1998 Does improved postoperative pain control improve sleep? Clinical Effectiveness in Nursing 2: 94–97

Cox K 1992 Quality of sleep in hospital settings. Doctoral dissertation, Faculteit der Gezondheidswetenschnappen, Rijksuniversiteit Limburg, Universitaire Pers, Maasstricht

Dodds E J 1980 Sleep well? A study of ward activity and nurse–patient interaction at night. M.Sc thesis, University of Surrey

Ellis B W, Dudley H A F 1976 Some aspects of sleep research in surgical stress. Journal of Psychosomatic Research 20: 303–308

Fehm H L, Benkowitsch R, Kern W, Fehm-Wolfsdorf G, Pauschinger P, Born J 1986 Influences of corticosteroids, dexamethasone, and hydrocortisone on sleep in humans. Neuropsychobiology 16: 198–204

Fife D, Rappaport E 1976 Noise and hospital stay. American Journal of Public Health 66: 680–681

Floyd J A 1984 Interaction between personal sleep–wake rhythms and psychiatric hospital rest–activity schedule. Nursing Research 33(5): 255–259

Fontaine D K 1989 Measurement of nocturnal sleep patterns in trauma patients. Heart and Lung 18: 402–410

Freed D L J 1975 Inadequate analgesia at night. Lancet 1: 519–520

Friess E, von Bardelben U, Wiedermann K, Lauer C J, Holsboer F 1994 Effects of pulsatile cortisol infusion on sleep-EEG and nocturnal growth hormone release in healthy men. Journal of Sleep Research 3: 73–79

Glyn C L, Lloyd J W, Folkard S 1976 The diurnal variation in the perception of pain. Proceedings of the Royal Society of Medicine 69: 369–372

Gronfier C, Luthringer R, Follenius M, Schaltenbrand N, Macher J P, Muzet A, Brandenberger G A 1996 A quantitative evaluation of the relationships between growth hormone secretion and delta wave electroencephalographic activity during normal sleep and after enrichment in delta waves. Sleep 19(10): 817–824

Grumet G W 1993 Pandemonium in the modern hospital. New England Journal of Medicine 328(6): 433–437

Hilakivi I 1987 Biogenic amines in the regulation of wakefulness and sleep. Medical Biology 65: 97–104

Hilton B A 1976 Quantity and quality of patients' sleep and sleep disturbing factors in a respiratory intensive care unit. Journal of Advanced Nursing 1(6): 453–468

Horne J 1988 Why we sleep. The functions of sleep in humans and other mammals. Oxford University Press, Oxford

Johns M W, Large A A, Masterton J P, Dudley H A F 1974 Sleep and delirium after open heart surgery. British Journal of Surgery 61(5): 377–381

Kavey N B, Altschuler K Z 1979 Sleep in herniorrhaphy patients. American Journal of Surgery 138: 682–687

Keefe M R 1987 Comparison of neonatal night-time sleep–wake patterns in nursery versus rooming-in environments. Nursing Research 36: 140–144

Kent S, Price M, Satinoff E 1988 Fever alters characteristics of sleep in rats. Physiology and Behaviour 44: 709–715

Knill R L, Moote C A, Skinner M I, Rose E A 1990 Anesthesia with abdominal surgery leads to intense REM sleep during the first post-operative week. Anesthesiology 73(1): 52–61

Lane R C, Fontaine D 1992 Sleep in the pediatric intensive care unit. Heart and Lung 21(3): 287

Lentz M J, Killien M G 1991 Are you sleeping? Sleep patterns during post-partum hospitalization. Journal of Perinatal and Neonatal Nursing 4(4): 30–38

MacFadyen U M, Oswald I, Lewis S A 1973 Starvation and human slow-wave sleep. Journal of Applied Physiology 35(3): 391–394

Mann N P, Hasddow R, Stokes L, Goodley S, Rutter N 1986 Effect of night and day on preterm infants in a newborn nursery: Randomised trial. British Medical Journal 293: 1265–1267

Marcus N 1995 Sleeping sickness. Nursing Standard 9(22): 56

Moldofsky H, Lue F A, Davidson J R, Gorczynski R 1989 The effects of sleep deprivation on human immune function. FASEB Journal 3: 1972–1977

Moote C A, Knill R L, Skinner M I, Rose E A 1989 Morphine disrupts sleep in a dose dependent fashion. Anesthesia and Analgesia 68: S200

Murphy F, Bentley S, Ellis B W, Dudley H 1977 Sleep deprivation in patients undergoing operations: a factor in the stress of surgery. British Medical Journal 2(610): 1521–1522

Ogilvie A J 1980 Sources and levels of noise on the ward at night. Nursing Times 76: 1363–1366

Orr W C, Stahl M L 1977 Sleep disturbances after open heart surgery. American Journal of Cardiology 39: 196–201

Pacini C M, Fitzpatrick J J 1982 Sleep patterns of hospitalized and non-hospitalized aged individuals. Journal of Gerontological Nursing 8: 327–323

Reimer M 1987 Sleep pattern disturbance: nursing interventions perceived by patients and their nurses as facilitating nocturnal sleep in hospital. In: McLane A M (ed) Classification of nursing diagnoses. Proceedings of the seventh conference, North American Nursing Diagnosis Association. C V Mosby, St Louis, pp 372–376

Rosenberg J, Wildschiødtz G, Pederson M H, von Jessen F, Kehlet H 1994 Late post-operative nocturnal episodic hypoxaemia and associated sleep pattern. British Journal of Anaesthesia 72: 145–150

Rosenberg-Adamsen S, Kehlet H, Dodds C, Rosenberg J 1996 Post-operative sleep disturbances: mechanisms and clinical implications. British Journal of Anaesthesia 76: 552–559

Royal College of Surgeons of England and the College of Anaesthetists 1990 Commission on the Provision of Surgical Services. Report of the Working Party on Pain After Surgery. London

Royal Commission on the National Health Service 1978 Patients' attitudes to the hospital service. HMSO, London

Scharf M B, Kales A, Bixler E O 1975 Readaptation to the sleep laboratory in insomniac subjects. Psychophysiology 12: 412–415

Schultz T J 1978 Synthesis of social surveys on noise annoyance. Journal of the Acoustic Society of America 64: 377–405

Shapiro C M, Flanigan M J 1993 ABC of sleep disorders. Function of sleep. British Medical Journal 306: 383–385

Sheely L C 1996 Sleep disturbances in hospitalized patients with cancer. Oncology Nursing Forum 23(1): 109–111

Soutar R L, Wilson J A 1986 Does hospital noise disturb patients? British Medical Journal 292: 305

Southwell M T, Wistow G 1995 Sleep in hospitals at night: are patients' needs being met? Journal of Advanced Nursing 21: 1101–1109

Stead W 1985 One awake, all awake! Nursing Mirror 160: 20–21

Walker B B 1972 The post-surgery heart patient: amount of uninterrupted time for sleep and rest during the first, second and third postoperative days in a teaching hospital. Nursing Research 21(2): 164–169

Williamson J W 1992 The effects of ocean sounds on sleep after coronary bypass graft surgery. American Journal of Critical Care 1(1): 91–97

Woods N 1972 Patterns of sleep in post-cardiotomy patients. Nursing Research 21: 347–352

Woolf C J 1995 How to hit pain before it hurts you. MRC News (Summer): 17–21

Yinnon A M, Ilan Y, Tadmor B, Altarescu G, Hersko C 1992 Quality of sleep in the medical department. British Journal of Clinical Practice 46: 88–91

Index

Note: page numbers in *italics* refer to figures and tables

Z